St. Augustine

O eternal truth, true love and beloved eternity.
You are my God.
To you do I sigh day and night.
When first I came to know you,
you drew me to yourself
so that I might see that there were things for me to see,
but that I myself was not yet ready to see them.
Meanwhile you overcame the weakness of my vision,
sending forth most strongly the beams of your light,
and I trembled at once with love and dread.

Late have I loved you,
O Beauty ever ancient, ever new,
late have I loved you!
You were within me, but I was outside,
and it was there that I searched for you.
In my unloveliness I plunged into the lovely things
which you created.
You were with me, but I was not with you.
Created things kept me from you;
yet if they had not been in you they would not have been at all.
You called,
you shouted,
and you broke through my deafness.
You flashed,
you shone,
and you dispelled my blindness.
You breathed your fragrance on me;
I drew in breath and now I pant for you.
I have tasted you, now I hunger and thirst for more.
You touched me,
and I burn for your peace.

Fasting Rediscovered

A GUIDE TO HEALTH AND WHOLENESS FOR YOUR BODY-SPIRIT

THOMAS RYAN

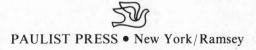

PAULIST PRESS • New York/Ramsey

Acknowledgments

I am deeply grateful to

George Fitzgerald, C.S.P. for believing in me and helping me give shape to a book that weds the spiritual, physiological, and social aspects of fasting;

the Sisters of the Congregation of Notre Dame of Montreal (especially Sr. Quinlan), Ton and Susan Zuydwijk, and Louise Forget for providing quiet space to write;

Ed Langlois, C.S.P., Marilyn Ryan, Kevin Munn, C.S.P., Elizabeth Richter, John P. Collins, C.S.P., Stuart B. Hill, Bill Noonan, C.S.P., and Michael Bernardin who read all parts of this manuscript and offered helpful suggestions;

Irene Sidorenko, Rose Mackie, Judy Roy and Virginia Farrelly who did the typing of the manuscript;

and Lou Pauly for his careful proofreading.
Thank you.

Library of Congress
Catalog Card Number: 80-81581

ISBN: 0-8091-2323-1

Published by Paulist Press
545 Island Road, Ramsey, N.J. 07446

Printed and bound in the
United States of America

Contents

DEDICATED

*to the Sisters of the Congregation of
Notre Dame of Montreal who are in the mother-
house infirmary:
your faith, hope, and quiet joy as you
live your own special kind of fast go right
to the heart of what makes Christian fasting
different from any other kind.*

1 *In Search of Lost Treasure*

> *What the parents throw away as useless,*
> *the children bring back as newfound treasure.*
> *What one generation discards, the other generation*
> *unearths and enshrines.*
>
> —Edward Farrell

Fasting Rediscovered

I fast to pull the loose ends together in my life.

I used to do a lot of things that were at cross-purposes with my own health and well-being. Fasting introduced me to a more genuinely life-supporting way to live.

Since I've been fasting, I'm more sensitive to what messages are coming from both my heart and my body.

About a year ago I began fasting one day a week. It's been the most settled, healthy, productive year of my life.

I was searching for a way of praying that went beyond words but which was at the same time both personal and did some good for my neighbor. Fasting has become the prayer of my whole self. My body, as well as my spirit, are involved in it.

More people are practicing voluntary fasting than we would ever guess. People who normally feel just "so-so" or. "O.K." are feeling abundantly alive. There is a new myth in the making: fasting is an effective means for realizing our full potential. People from all ages and backgrounds are fasting: athletes, musicians, students, teachers, union leaders, clergy, medical professionals, artists, construction workers, designers, writers, photographers, secretaries, actors, bus drivers and store managers. The rediscovery of fasting is like a new great awakening that is cutting across all societal lines and claiming followers from every sector of human experience.

Why are they fasting? There are several reasons, though not all of them motivate every person who fasts. Perhaps the reason that is most often present as a motivational factor is that of body-ecology. We are becoming much more aware of a very real wisdom and intelligence operating in our body processes. Many people are fasting simply to give their physical self a rest, a holiday. The body is constantly absorbed in the work of digesting food, metabolizing it into energy, and eliminating the waste materials. To go without eating from time to time is to reward our body-selves with the same kind of vacation that we give our minds after we've been working hard at reading or writing. Our bodies have lots of tasks to accomplish: digestion, elimination, fighting diseases, replenishing worn-out cells, and rejuvenating the blood. Of all these, one of the most taxing is digestion. When we stop putting food into the body for a time, some of the other important internal concerns receive more attention. Fasting, in short, gives the body a chance to renew itself. It is a time in which the body burns its rubbish. It's like house-cleaning day.

Our era is seeing a consciousness-raising in the area of personal health. Witness the "Thank You For Not Smoking" buttons, the proliferation of health-food stores, and the omnipresent joggers. It shouldn't come as surprising, then, that as people rediscover that fasting is healthy, more and more have been interested in trying it and want to know more about it.

Dr. Yuri Nikolayev, who has been conducting controlled hunger experiments at the Moscow Research Institute of Psychiatry, shared these comments on fasting by an unidentified man who has practiced regular fasting for fifty years. His comments appear in Allan Cott's *Fasting: The Ultimate Diet*, and express the kind of focus on personal health that is motivating many people to fast today:

> In my opinion, the biggest discovery of our time is the ability to make oneself younger—physically, mentally, and spiritually—through rational fasting. With the help of fasting one can forget his age and thus prevent the processes of premature aging. I am 85 years old and proud of my agility. I can easily do yoga exercises standing on my head. Few people my age are able to do such exercises. I eat twice a day and never between meals. Every week I fast for 24 hours and three or four times a year for

6

seven to ten days at a time . . . To be strong and healthy and to enjoy it—one has to work. . . . But remember, only you can work for your health! You cannot buy it and nobody will give it to you. I am in perfect health and feel energetic, all because I learned nature's laws and follow them. Fasting is the key to health; it purifies every cell in the body. I am sure that 99 percent of the sick people suffer because of improper nourishment. People simply do not understand that they litter the body by many unnatural foods, and—because of this—poisonous substances are collected in the body. If you are interested in being in good physical and mental health and increasing vitality, start to work for this today *with nature*, not against her.

Another major reason underlying the fasting of many today is that they are experiencing it as an aid to self-transcendence, to going beyond themselves. Tennessee Williams wrote of his own discovery in this regard in his autobiography, *Memoirs*. After three days without food as a young man he noted that "God or somebody drops in on you invisibly and painlessly injects you with a sedation so that you find yourself drifting into a curiously and absolutely inexplicably peaceful condition, and this condition is ideal for meditation on things past and passing and to come, in just that sequence."

Many people who would describe themselves as "religious" and who at one time practiced fasting and/or abstinence have dropped it, perhaps because at some point it began to feel like a rote discipline, a negative practice, something required by law but without consciously perceived purpose or value. An article in the *Christian Century* entitled "For God's Sake, Fast For Your Own Sake!" stated that even if your faith can't motivate you to do it, it's still worth doing!

Health and Wholeness

Not much has been done by way of books or articles that help people to integrate the physical and the spiritual benefits of fasting. It doesn't have to be either-or. It can and should be both, because we are not just bodies and we are not just spirits. We are embodied spirits. Enspirited flesh. What is good for me physically is good for me. And what is good for me spiritually is good for me. There's only one "I" to which it all comes back. This holistic approach is my perspective throughout this book; it underlies both the theological and physiological sections.

"Holism" was first set forth in a dialogue with Darwinian evolutionists in a book called *Holism and Evolution* by the Right Honorable J.C. Smuts. He said:

> From this new viewpoint a re-survey will be made relating to matter, life, and mind, and an attempt will be made to reach the fundamental unity and continuity which underlie and connect all three. We shall thus come to see all three as connected steps in the same great Process. . . .

The goal of his book was to give "a new interpretation of Nature wherein Matter, Life and Mind, so far from being discontinuous and disparate will appear as a more or less connected progressive series of the same great Process." For his time, it was a new viewpoint, because the current scientific and philosophical thought did not recognize such a fundamental continuity in the human person.

Today, "psychosomatic" is a household word. We get sick and a colleague asks us if we've been feeling a lot of stress lately. The holistic approach has worked its way down from the scientific circles to the layman in the streets where the body-spirit unity of which it speaks is now generally accepted as "the way things are." Kurt Goldstein, writing in the late 1930's, gave further momentum to Smuts' insight in a book called *Human Nature in the Light of Psychopathology*. He said:

> . . . one has to consider each single symptom in terms of its functional significance for the total personality . . . Thus it is obviously necessary for the physician to know *the organism as a whole*, the total personality of his patient . . . The whole organism, the individual human being, becomes the center of interest.

The medical and social sciences today accept the holistic approach as valid and true. We are not "two things," i.e., a body *and* a soul. We are one seamless multidimensional person. The most positive experience I ever had with any doctor came at a time when I had just been diagnosed as having mononucleosis. He took me into a

8

little room off the corridor and talked with me about my *life*—its demands, tensions and anxieties. We talked about work and play, fatigue and rest. When I walked out of there, I felt as though I understood, in terms of my whole life at that time, why I had been sick. He responded to me holistically.

My physical self is not merely an object with which I am confronted; it is something which I myself *am*. The pleasure and pain of my body are *my* pleasure and pain. I can never distinguish myself adequately from my body; I am the particular person I am precisely on account of my bodily individuation. And my human spirit reaches its full concrete reality only in its relation to my body, which is its expression, its way of being "there." When Pascal said "man is only what he is by being thus greater than himself," he was talking about spirit. The human spirit is our most essential dimension because it is the way we are able to open constantly outward beyond ourselves.

The coexistence of our body-spirit is not without tension, however. Our bodily nature limits us in space and time; it prevents us from expressing ourselves fully, as every thinker, lover and artist has experienced. It absorbs energies in the effort to speak that should really be devoted to the actual statement. This dialectical situation affects every happening of everyday life, but it is most apparent in the supreme events of eros and death. At these pre-eminent moments the temptation to which we are exposed by this tension is displayed most clearly. It is the temptation to give up the effort of unification and to live on two different planes. It is the temptation to restrict oneself to any one of the two regions: either a corporeal existence hostile to the spirit, or a spiritual existence filled with hatred of the body.

To succumb to the temptation is equal to ceasing to be human. The truth is that the fluid dialectical relationship of unity and opposition within our embodied spirit can neither be transcended nor dissolved.

This discussion of fasting, therefore, goes forward with its focus on both our physical and our spiritual good. As a friend exclaimed when she heard I was working on this book: "I've read all the books on fasting in the health-food stores, and there's nothing I know of that deals with it as a religious act in a faith context. If you can integrate that with the physiological considerations and put the two out there together to be taken as one whole, you'll be making a real contribution."

That, in any case, is the objective: to integrate "the two" and present them as one unified concern. Hence the sub-title:*A Guide to Health and Wholeness For Your Body-Spirit.*

Of Pleasure and Temperance

Pat Dominic is a university graduate student. He discovered fasting a few years ago.

My first experience with fasting was a Day of Fast for World Hunger sponsored by the university campus ministry. It was the first time I had ever gone a whole day without food. There was a prayer vigil that evening at which people gave the money which they would have spent on food that day. Half of it went to the neighborhood agency, and the other half to Bread For the World. I remember that I had a headache when I went home that evening, but I was even more aware that something had touched my heart. I had these intimations of a power in fasting that I wanted to know more about.

A couple of months later, I saw a blurb in the campus paper about a Lenten Bible Study series called "The Adventure of Fasting" to be held at the Newman Center. I was struck by that title. My one day fasting experience had been a novel and a good experience, but not exactly what I would call an "adventure."

Anyway, I bit. And since then, well, I guess you could say I've been hooked . . . .

A friend of mine has this saying which he uses as a joke whenever it suits his purposes: "Moderation in all things— including moderation!" I had never thought about moderation or temperance more seriously than that.

To me, temperance suggested the Women's Temperance League or something. Some old maid going around trying to prevent others from enjoying food or drink or card-playing or sex. The whole notion of Temperance was *against* (it didn't matter what)!

I must admit, I got my head turned around on a lot of things in that Bible Study. We did a survey of all the passages on fasting and talked a lot about its human roots in moderation and temperance. I started to develop a positive set of associations around those words. . . .

A couple of other notions that were fresh for me were that fasting is a way of communicating with God and a way of caring for God's personal gift to us: ourselves.

I started fasting a day a week, using just water, and have been doing that for about a year now. I'd be hard put to tell you what a qualitative difference has emerged in my life—in all its aspects!

Fasting has become like sending God a message: sometimes the message is "I want to find you in all the clutter in my life"; at other times it's "I really want you to help this person"; at still other times it's "I'm sorry" or "I need a rest." It's a very real message, written in "body-language." While fasting comes from the heart, I've also come to see it as the prayer of the body.

And that's another thing: since I've been fasting regularly, I haven't been sick. not even a cold (knock on wood!). I'm not trying to say fasting is the only reason—I'm sure there are others, too; but there's no question in my mind that it's *one* of the reasons. I really have never felt better.

I don't like to make long-term projections because they usually end up being rash and not coming true anyhow, but I feel quite secure in making an exception in this case: I'm going to be fasting regularly for the rest of my life. Something's been coming through in my experience that feels so right, and I know deep inside me I'm on to something very big.

What comes through in Pat's "witness" is not just fasting as a "body-thing" or fasting just as a "religious-thing." The two appear in relationship to each other, integrated into the overall unity of his life.

The key to this harmonious integration, I believe, appears in his reference to temperance and moderation. This is the place from which the project of developing a holistic vision of fasting's benefits must begin: with an appreciation of the virtue of temperance. One of the best discussions I have ever come across on the subject is in Walter Farrell's *A Companion to the Summa*. Temperance is like a chain with a hook on each end: one end attaches to physiological health, the other end attaches to spiritual health. The chain goes out in both directions and links the two because temperance has implications for the health and wholeness of my embodied spirit taken as a whole.

Temperance is the genus, fasting the species; temperance is a game, fasting the player; temperance is the book, fasting the chapter. An appreciation of temperance's role in the development of a healthy, happy, human person is the background for our consideration of fasting. The discussion will take place from the perspective of Christian faith.

11

Temperance relates directly to pleasure. A few pages on the meaning of pleasure may seem like an unnecessary digression in a book on fasting. It's not. Far from being a roundabout country road, it's an interstate highway that is the most direct route to where we're going, precisely because the immediate visceral response of many people to the mere word "fasting" is: "Ugh—that wouldn't be pleasurable."

A father of three remarked to me recently that he is having difficulty interesting his youngest daughter in accompanying the family to church. "Why should I do that," she said, "that's no fun." The father's reflection was that "our society is raising a generation of pleasure-junkies. 'Will it feel good?' is the criterion against which everything is judged."

The place and meaning of pleasure in our lives is, then, an important preliminary consideration. Especially when dealing with a subject that may have first-level negative associations by virtue of being perceived as "no fun." What those who try fasting are surprised to learn is that there is a deep and abiding sense of pleasure in it—the pleasure that comes with both feeling remarkably healthy and sensing a growing intimacy with the Lord. There is immense pleasure in a balanced and centered life.

Temperance essentially has to do with balance. To begin with, there is a lack of balance in our general thinking about temperance. The very word calls to mind the fanatical reformer or tavern brawls. It is not only easy to embrace an extreme, there is a guarantee of assurance about it. There will always be applause for the extremist no matter which extreme he embraces, and there will always be a double opposition in store for the person who rejects both extremes. The medium of reason often seems an uncolorful, ordinary manner of procedure. Actually, to embrace either extreme means a lack of balance.

This virtue of balance relates to all the pleasures whose allure may draw us off the course of moderating reason. One of the obvious reasons why temperance is not a popular notion today is that our society has, as noted above by my friend, an incredible hang-up with pleasure. This hang-up affects society even as influenced by Christianity, whose stand on pleasure ought to have been made perfectly clear by the miracle of Cana and by the constant and pervasive use of sexual imagery in Christian sacred writings. The Christian who feels guilty when she enjoys a glass of good red wine or the body of her man is not a good Christian.

Enjoyment and pleasure have been viewed with great suspicion by most of the world's major religions. With the exception of Christianity, Judaism, and Islam, the human person is viewed as a spirit trapped in a body. The spirit is good, the body is evil. Pleasure and enjoyment are bodily functions and therefore contribute to the imprisonment of the spirit. The Christian response to this is that we are not just a trapped spirit, but enspirited flesh, all of which has been redeemed. Jesus attended feasts, drank wine, and worked a miracle to prevent a party from collapsing. There is more sexual imagery in our sacred books than that of any other religion. The notion that pleasure is, if not evil, at least to be distrusted, has a pre-Christian origin. It is a notion that has survived despite Christian doctrine and to some extent has even prevented Christians from seeing the implications of their own doctrine.

Temperance is not the puritanical enemy of pleasure; its goal is not repression or inhibition. It does not frown on all that is attractive in life. Rather than attacking sense pleasures, it guarantees them. It is a good habit proclaiming present and past mastery of reason, protecting, as well as predicting, the humanity of future actions. It is interested in safeguarding the happy medium of reason which is the absolutely essential condition for peace and progress in human life. It insists on the full freedom that can be given only by intelligent control.

Michael Bernadin is the Director for the Montreal Society for Emotionally Disturbed Children. When he feels that certain delicate inner focus becoming blurred, he tempers the bombardment of stimuli with fasting. It's a form of temperance in his life:

When my life is going too fast, I tend to be mentally all over the place, and not sensitive enough to the person or event that is present right now. When I fast, I listen better, I'm clearer in what I say—perhaps because it's more peaceful inside myself. Fasting represents for me a respite from the overstimulations of life, whether it be from auditory, visual, or food sources.

I fast to pull the loose threads together in my life—it's a movement within. When I'm in touch with what's within, I find I'm in tune with what's without. Some people call it "being filled with the Holy Spirit"; others, being "in tune with the universe." The "Holy Spirit" isn't part of my frequent vocabulary, but whatever words people use, I feel the reality being described is much the same.

13

As I've been fasting periodically during the past three years, I've realized that it works on more levels than one, and I find that all the aspects of my life just flow better.

For Michael, fasting is like the fine-tuning knob on a stereo, enabling him to receive the signals being transmitted in his direction with greater clarity, and to give clearer messages himself. A day characterized by such communication is a satisfying day. Such satisfaction, found amidst the rigors of one's work, is a deep and quiet pleasure—a pleasure born of temperance.

There is a sense of pleasure necessarily and naturally connected with the very use of the necessities of life. Temperance does not—cannot—touch that pleasure. Pleasure is simply the experience that we have when we come into physical contact with the enjoyable aspects of our environment. To reject or repress pleasure is to deny either the goodness of our bodiliness or the goodness of the world with which we come into contact. In the Christian tradition, both alternatives are untenable. Temperance does not blast out any part of our nature; it does not ask that we keep a few drops of castor oil on our tongue all the time to counteract the natural pleasure of eating. It insists on moderation in those things that add to the essential pleasure, that make the natural use a still greater source of pleasure.

Physical pleasure is essentially an ecstatic experience and as such it takes us out of ourselves and forces us to be aware of the reality beyond ourselves and to acknowledge that that reality is good. However minor or intense our pleasures may be, they represent rewarding contacts with external reality and demand that we abandon our attempts to isolate ourselves inside the walls of our own intellectuality and cut ourselves off from all contact with the physical world.

Pleasure, of course, can become selfish, but at root it is an antidote to selfishness because it entices us to share our bodies and ourselves with the rest of the world. When pleasure pours in and opens us up to the world (even if we do not want to be so opened), our selfishness, our narrowness, our cynicism are overwhelmed.

The idea that ecstasy takes us out of ourselves and opens us up to others in love and faith and hope is by no means a Christian monopoly, but the idea that the union between God and his people is a pleasurable union comparable to marriage *is* uniquely Christian.

The Christian's critical question is not the legitimacy of pleasure or enjoyment, but rather the coordination of pleasure with the other

14

goals of human life. It is precisely here that we must come to grips with a fundamental principle of human experience: limitation is essential for the integration of the personality. This is the birthplace of temperance as virtue. Pleasure must be limited if it is to be enjoyed. Limitation means that pleasure must be seen in the context of one's whole life project. Too many times in our libertarian era limitation of any kind has been seen as stunting, stifling, and dehumanizing.

. The athlete in training is not inhuman because she limits her social engagements. The invalid recovering from a severe fever is not condemning food when he abstains from corned beef and cabbage. The monk dedicated to contemplation has an entirely different diet than the brawny bricklayer.

Temperance is not empty-headed. It is filled with common sense. It is a quality of beauty because the very essence of beauty is proportion. And temperance has as its striking note precisely that of moderation, of order, of proportion. It has an air of tranquility about it, like the beauty of a calm sea, a Vermont valley farm seen from a mountain top, or a child's face immediately after a bath. Temperance is an intensely personal virtue, as beauty is an intensely personal thing. Yet it is a constant inspiration to others, as beauty always is. It is the refreshing touch of the breath of God's order.

There is always an implication of immaturity in sins of intemperance; an insistence that we pay as little attention to reason as an adolescent pays to the wisdom of experience; a contention that we have no more possibility of putting order in our lives than has a child as yet incapable of reasoning. Intemperance argues, in other words, that human nature cannot take care of itself, cannot induce order, proportion, moderation in its own house.

And that is no less than a denial to human nature of the claim it has for dignity and self-respect: the command of our own lives. The human individual is thus robbed of that personal responsibility, that personal control, that personal reward or punishment that is wrapped up with the inherent dignity of human freedom. As Leon Bloy wrote, "Our freedom is God's respect for us."

There are reasons for why we choose slavery over mastery. Perhaps the most outstanding is the difficult condition attached to temperance, that is, the condition of battle. It is a peculiarly difficult battle, for its end is not to destroy or break the power of an opponent, but to keep intact and working together all the power and energy of the different "interest groups." Reason, if it is to reign at all, must reign as a constitutional monarch, granting full representation to both the animal and the mystic in us.

The appeal of mastery to our nature is constant and profound, precisely because we were made to exercise it. It was not mistaken strategy that moved the devil to offer Eve the prospect of becoming like God. His appeal was to nothing less than complete dominion, perfect mastery. Our nature responds to the goal for which it was created; that is why the prospect of mastery sets us afire. What is human history but a series of attempts in every age to rise again to the bait of mastery?

The subject for mastery in this case is ourselves. The capacity for mastery is not only presumed, it is given and revealed in the Spirit of Jesus Christ who "is with us for all days" and who has "already overcome the world." Temperance, our response to the urging of the Holy Spirit to give a God-intended proportion to our lives, is like an aqueduct that carries the water of health, inner peace, and tranquillity.

The Christian church today, as indeed in all days, is the champion of temperance. Mocked in one age as the mother of looseness, ungodliness, frivolity and pleasure, derided in another age as the narrow, dour-faced advocate of conservatism, rigidity, prudishness and angelism, she is in fact none of these things: She is the champion of humanity; insisting on beauty in human life, insisting now as always that we *are* body as well as spirit. She stands by the fundamental truth that we are equipped for, by virtue of God's grace, and capable of ordering our own lives creatively and constructively. She continues to urge us to fulfill God's dream for us, and to refuse to give it up whatever the sacrifice demands, because she knows that the human person cannot cease to be master without at the same time ceasing to be human. "Be fruitful, multiply, fill the earth, and subdue it" (Genesis 1:22).

Any discussion of fasting that wants to go forward simultaneously on the levels of physical health and spiritual growth needs two cornerstones. The first is, hopefully, in place: an appreciative grasp of the meaning of and place for temperance in modern life. We are now ready for the second cornerstone—a basic comprehension of the meaning of Christian asceticism—to be set in place. After that, our full attention can be brought to bear upon fasting itself.

Christian Asceticism

Christian asceticism originated in the following observation dear to the Fathers of the Church and found in almost identical terms in the works of Clement of Alexandria and St. Augustine: "The man who lets himself do everything that is allowed will very soon become slack and do what is not allowed." Asceticism's link with temperance is obvious and strong.

The noted author, theologian, and spiritual director George A. Maloney observes that if today many basically good Christian people do not have a feeling of being alive and human (which is to say, saintly), the reason may be the exaggerated misunderstandings coming down through the centuries that are attached to two venerable words in the Christian tradition: asceticism and mysticism. Mysticism essentially relates to living with the awareness of God's presence; and asceticism essentially relates to any conscious practice that helps us move from a self-centering life to a God-centering life. Both have been, in the constant interpretation of the faith, inseparable elements in the development of a totally Christian life.

We would be fools not to be aware of the gulf between the Christian ideal and the condition of society today. The competition for the human spirit is an all-out one with no holds barred. Concerns of the spirit are almost smothered by the superficial until our milieu has become a desert with only a trickle of living water to refresh weary humanity. As Saudi Arabia's late King Ibn Saud once said, "In my youth I met God in the desert, and God gave me the secret of success. To me everything is opportunity, even an obstacle." The only way to meet the competition of present-day living is to muster an increase of spiritual energy. In other words, a healthy and realistic asceticism.

Since fasting is a Christian asceticism, it is pertinent for us to get a clear understanding of what asceticism means, why ascetical practices developed, and what purpose and application they have in our lives today.

Asceticism has generally referred, in Christian writings, to the deliberate and persevering endeavor of the Christian to attain full human development, which is the same as "Christian perfection." From the viewpoint of faith, we cannot know what human development is outside of Jesus. In other words, anthropology or the study of humanness becomes Christology or the study of Christ, because it is only in Christ that we find fully realized the farther reaches of our human nature. To do anthropology in that context is also to do theology. Full humanness becomes Christhood. Or, full human development Christian perfection.

In practice there are a great many obstacles to such an endeavor: the tension/conflict between our body and spirit dimensions, our

17

own inner weaknesses, and sinful influences from outside ourselves. It necessarily means a struggle, self-denial and a letting-go of certain things which may be perfectly good in and of themselves. Hence the word ascetics, which really means exercise, has acquired a special meaning of exertion, struggle and abstinence.

The practices or exercises of the Christian life that come under the heading "ascetical" should always be considered as a means and a help to overcome all obstacles that prevent the Christian from loving God and neighbor. They have both a negative and positive side. The negative side concerns *metanoia*, or conversion: the turning away from evil, from sinful inclination and desires. The positive side implies a loving turning toward God and one's neighbor, the practice of moral principles and virtues, restoration of the sin-disturbed inner order, the dominance of selfless love. The entire process involves a cleansing of the heart, inward recollection and composure, and a growing experience of God and of union with him.

The truly fundamental Christian asceticism or "exercise" is undoubtedly faith, which is of course primarily a gift of God. But God, who makes himself known in his revelation and in our hearts, must be answered not once but every day. This "exercise," this acceptance of the grace of faith, this "yes" to God who is revealing himself, not only gives fulfillment and enlightenment, but is also essentially an act of self-denial. In faith we accept the mystery of God which for us is unfathomable and impenetrable, and we give ourselves trustingly to God without seeing what we have been promised. We thus let go of any *isolated* attempt on our own to find the meaning of our own existence, of the world in general and its history. Guided by our faith in him who has promised eternal life, we are constantly fighting to transcend ourselves, to let go of ourselves. This is the very basis of our asceticism. One might call it the asceticism of faith, the exercise of self-surrender to almighty God whom one cannot see, whose judgments are unsearchable, and whose ways are inscrutable.

The friend who shared the following thoughts said "it's hard to get too personal about your ascetical practices in public; I'd prefer this to be anonymous." So be it. His reflections stand by themselves as an example of the above:

I think fasting is part of the Christian life. Jesus fasted, and said his followers would also fast when he was gone.

Fasting is a way of deepening dependency, and thus if embarked upon in faith can deepen our dependency upon God.

It helps to remind me that I am a creature, totally dependent upon God for everything.

Fasting is also an act of worship for me. It's giving God my body more totally. By fasting I say to him, "My body has come from you. Your will is my basic food and drink. May I always use my body for your service and not in any way for selfishness."

Unfortunately, there is a tendency for the very word *asceticism* to receive a negative judgment in the courtroom of the modern mind. "Asceticism," in the minds of most people only vaguely familiar with its meaning, projects an ideal of religion that is a throwback to the self-sacrificing practices of the monastic era where religious leaders called for separation from the world. In contemporary judgment, such a withdrawal is unhealthy; consequently the word asceticism fell into disrepute, associated as it was with anachronistic customs and excessive practices. This reaction left a void that in turn led to a malaise in the spiritual life.

Ascetical practices that had become cut off from their life-giving source and which had become ends in themselves (e.g., the Friday abstinence from meat, observed till recently by Roman Catholics) have been repudiated in the last twenty years. Many ascetical practices were judged to be several times removed from the historical, cultural, and individual context from which they had derived their meaning, and were dropped as incompatible with the contemporary world.

Whatever new or renewed shapes it takes, Christian asceticism has to avoid the kind of one-sidedness, suspicion and curtailment that it has met with at times in the traditional attitude toward the body, sex, marriage and "worldly" matters in general. It must approach the human person as an embodied spirit living in the world, for the grace of God speaks to the whole person in all his or her aspects.

Thus, all anthropological disciplines have a place in Christian asceticism: physiology, psychology, sociology, etc., as well as the various ways of being woman or man and developing as a human person: individual and social aspects, especially the polarity and meeting of the sexes, marriage and celibacy; property and poverty, work, vocation, political action; age, the course of life, and so on. All these are the components that must be included in one's consideration if one is to arrive at an asceticism suitably adapted to an individual's sex, psychology and character, age, state of maturity,

19

status, environment and task. Hence, the variability of Christian asceticism, according to the demands of one's vocation and the concrete situation.

One senses a ripeness today for a return to Christian asceticism properly understood: not as an end in itself, but as a means of simplifying life so as to be more responsive to the intimations of grace. The recurring problem with ascetical practices has always been a confusion of the means and the end. There is always the danger of aiming at a pious achievement for its own sake and of making ourselves and our own personal perfection the center of religious effort.

As we try to rediscover the value of an ascetical practice like fasting, the challenge will be to keep straight in our own understanding that fasting as a religious act is not an end in itself, but is always for the purpose of helping us deepen our experience of God and our unity with God.

Arlene Becker lives and works in "the marketplace" in Ottawa, Ontario. She speaks of the reason why she fasts:

> I try to fast once a week for twenty-four hours and during the week one or two half days, meaning from evening one day to noon the next day. The only reason in my life for fasting is for the sake of love and living the Gospel.
>
> The thing I keep in mind most when fasting is that fasting is a matter of FAITH and OBEDIENCE. It is not something I would do naturally except perhaps for health reasons. But fasting as a Christian means to me taking a step in faith and obeying the word of God.
>
> Fasting has a depth of effects. One grows into fasting and grows into the effects of fasting. There is mystery in fasting which I believe will be more and more revealed simply through faithfulness to fasting. And yet if I learn nothing else about fasting, what I have learned is enough reason to do it till the end.
>
> One main discovery: fasting proves that God is the deepest part of us— He is in fact at the bottom of an empty stomach, so to speak. He is deeper than food and our desire for food. His love creates, sustains, and redeems us.
>
> To me fasting is simply a part of the commandment to love. It's purpose is love and its fruit is love. In obeying the word of God to fast I've discovered my prayers for others carry more love—and the power of love heals, blesses and brings life.

Fasting, first of all, leads one to experience a new dimension of God's love which is expressed in the words of Scripture: "I am the bread of life." God is our creator, our redeemer, our sustainer. And secondly, it is an expression of love for others: prayer with fasting increases our love for others.

Reclaiming Our Ascetical Tradition

Recent years have seen the emergence of personal-growth movements and with it the act of fasting as a valued regimen for their members. Most of these movements draw heavily upon the tradition and wisdom of Eastern religions and stress the combining of fasting and meditation as a means of achieving higher consciousness and awareness.

There is much that is valuable from these sources that we should be open to and gratefully receive, but have we turned so fully toward the East that we are no longer open to or aware of the riches in our own spiritual traditions?

The undeniable phenomenon of young Christians of every denomination rushing after new forms of spirituality among non-Christian sects should be a clear indicator for us to revisit our tradition.

We have seen the newspaper ads for Transcendental Meditation and probably know someone who practices it. We have seen a group of young adults beating a drum and shaking a tambourine to a Hare Krishna chant on a street corner on in an airport. We may have read *The Zen of Motorcycle Racing* or *The Zen of Running*. And chances are someone on our block knows where the Yogi's Hashram is on the local university campus. These Eastern methods of contacting the deepest Ground of our Being are being used by believers and nonbelievers alike. They have enriched the lives of many.

It is not the fact that many Christians have become enthusiastic participants in the psychic and spiritual benefits of TM, Yoga, and Zen that poses the question. It is that they have left their own religion with its liturgies and devotions and practices to do so.

Why do people leave the Christian faith only to end up a few years down the pike subscribing to the teachings of the latest Guru or Swami or Divine Master? Why do the same men and women who not so long ago dismissed priests and nuns, ministers and monks as only remotely relevant, now sit at the feet of robed Gurus or probe the mystic mantras of Krishna consciousness?

21

Perhaps because they were never really put in touch with the Divine Master of Christianity, and so it is a new and exciting thing to sit at the feet of anyone who seems to know something about the spiritual life. It is painful for us in the "mainline" churches to admit it—especially we "religious professionals"—but apparently many people are so starved for communication with God that they find the spirituality of other religious traditions watering their souls like springs in the desert.

In the consumption-oriented Western world and the atheistic-based Communist world, the message has been that sensible, material realities are the only realities worth knowing. While it is true that each era breeds its own kind of problems, it is also true that it develops its own mechanisms for balancing the excesses. Thus, the young today, pampered by an affluent society, have turned to Eastern religions in search of "a way" that will teach them discipline and help them discover realities discernible only to the "inner senses."

Perhaps the time has come when Christians old and young are ready to look again at ascetical practices that were observed in their earlier years and which were swept away. The experience of the shallowness of Western materialism's overindulgence has not been without its lesson for us. We are like a person who, sated with food to the point of discomfort, decides that it may feel better not to eat so much.

We are ready to fast. A sign of the Holy Spirit's presence in our lives is that something in our deepest selves is telling us to go against the conditioning of our consumerist society, to take a stand at odds with the ways of the culture of our time in history. The same Spirit is moving in us who moved in Jesus, telling him to go against the conditioning of a society that bid him speak politely when arguing with the Scribes and Pharisees, that bid him to keep a dignified distance from Mary Magdalene and the Samaritan woman, that bid him ignore the businessmen in the temple instead of throwing them out. Our deepest selves, enlightened by the Spirit of Jesus, may sometimes inspire us to walk upstream against the current, too, albeit in less dramatic daily situations.

Mary Jane Reed is a wife and mother to five children. She and her husband Bob are Mormons and live in Chicago. She tells of the extra effort and struggle involved in maintaining the practice of fasting:

I was introduced to fasting when we were investigating the Church.* I couldn't imagine going twenty-four hours without food or liquids—Bob even less so. It was quite a discovery to find how readily the body can do this and how good one feels. The fast offering is related to the welfare services of the Church, but its purpose is also for individual spiritual growth. That involves self-discipline and humility. There is also an emphasis on making that twenty-four-hour period a very spiritual one— being more reflective, and engaging in activities that would foster this.

In addition, it is very common for members to fast at other times on their own when there is something in their lives that is a special matter of prayer, be it petition or thanksgiving or confirmation of a decision, etc. Fasting and prayer just go together. You often hear people say—"I'll have to fast over that"—or if you're undertaking a big project whether at work, church or home, or you are beginning a new calling or job responsibility—you really wouldn't be sincere in your desire for the Lord's guidance and support if you didn't fast for that spiritual strength as well as pray.

In the meantime Bob encountered a book entitled *Fasting Can Save Your Life*—not a very readable book, but it deals with how fasting has alleviated specific illnesses and gives case histories. Since he has a lot of allergies he thought this might be a help. Thus we were introduced to fasting as a means of cleansing the body. He saw this book at a health-food store while making a sales call one day.

Though I haven't been very successful in consistently following a program of fasting for 1-2 days per week and eating only natural foods—I did fast for 7½ days once with only distilled water with lemon juice and honey to drink, when needed. It's an exhilarating feeling, and I couldn't believe how easy it was. I did notice that my senses were more acute,

---

*"A proper fast-day observance consists of abstaining from food and drink for two consecutive meals, attending the fast and testimony meeting, and making a generous offering to the bishop for the care of those in need. A minimum fast offering is defined as the equivalent of two meals." (*Mormon General Handbook of Instructions*, 1968, p. 40.)

especially smell. I felt more in control of *everything*. I seemed to always have a perspective on things so that an individual crisis did not get me down. I could deal with it calmly as though I were living in an environment removed from the bustle of things around me. Why did I do it? I just wanted to see what it would be like to fast and how long I could do it.

It would appear that there are two types of fasting—fasting for spiritual purposes and fasting for health. However, in *Doctrine and Covenants* (one of the Mormon's sacred books) we are told that the Lord says that He gives no law that is not spiritual. In other words, in the Word of Wisdom when we are told what kinds of foods to eat and to avoid, that's not a physical but a spiritual law, too. So even fasting for health becomes a spiritual fast. It's a commitment to a way of life, one that would surely require a great deal of self-discipline—especially when what's happening around you isn't supportive of it.

Fasting is then a program not only of health, but also of self-discipline—which naturally develops the "inner man." There is something special about fasting in that it does seem to remove you a step from the world around you and put you in touch with a more spiritual realm. I feel like I can't really live without it—or I should say progress without it. The Savior says he teaches us "precept by precept, line upon line," gives us "milk before meat"—he says "let those who have ears to hear let them hear . . . eyes to see, let them see." I think it's a necessary step in perfecting ourselves and becoming like the Savior. I don't think there's a substitute for what it has to offer.

I probably sound like I'm really on top of everything. Not quite! I feel that I've made a most valuable discovery, I'm deeply convinced of *fasting*, natural eating, and physical fitness as a way of life. While my execution is not as consistent as I'd like, I do have the satisfaction of knowing that I have a plan. Between the demands of husband, home, daughters, day-care children, and church, I feel like I'm barely holding it together sometimes. But a program of fasting and right eating, along with daily scripture study and regular journal entries, represents for me the strength to see it all through. It takes a great deal of concentration. Yet, establishing this in the midst of present demands sets up a certain conflict as both require concentration of different types, simultaneously. So most of

the time, I feel that I've progressed a step, and fallen back two—
but I keep on going.

It's a constant challenge to keep it up—it seems there's
much less progress than when I was pre-children, pre-home
owner, pre-husband, because I was more "in control" of my life
then. So much of my life now becomes determined by these
other circumstances—e.g., husband wants to go to bed earlier
or get up later than you might so you need to seek another time
for private prayer or study; when you get the housework done
and have some "free time," the children need some attention;
husband and children may not want to eat what you are so it's
two meal preparations when you can barely get one done.
Proper planning and organizing would alleviate a lot of this,
but let's face it, sometimes you're just so bone-weary and
emotionally fatigued that it's easier to just "hang it all up." So
progress isn't always a steady line forward! But I do feel the
Savior is teaching me this principle now. It's always been
around; I'm just "hearing" and "seeing" it now—it's the next
"line" and "precept" I need to know and implement to build
toward perfection and realize the person I really am.

The Meaning of Discipleship

If we are genuinely interested in becoming disciples of the Lord,
we will have to make room within our world view for a healthy sense
of asceticism. For being a disciple means to follow a truth or a person
who is a bearer of truth. To know myself as God's servant. To take
into account what he wishes me to do in this world. To really care
about myself and others.

The true disciple engages in the noblest of tasks: to unfold the
masterpiece of God's creation—the human person. Discipline, from
the same root as "disciple," far from being a stern master, is a gentle
mode of love. Adrian Van Kaam and Susan Muto express it with a
sensitive parallel:

Think how appalled we would be if our favorite artist, painting
a fine landscape, suddenly began to daub his canvas at random
because he became bored and disinterested. As regrettable is
our refusal to follow the inner call to be our best selves. Lack of
discipline, in this case, clearly retards our growth ... Discipline

25

is that which draws the artist to complete his picture or the poet to devote himself untiringly to the word.

The deepest meaning of discipleship comes into focus when we reflect upon the mysteries of Jesus' life. His death and resurrection become the path we must follow. Even before that paschal event, he preached the mystery of dying in order that life might flourish. He looked at the fig tree and observed that it must be pruned so new leaves could grow. He noted that the seed dropped into the earth must die if it is to bear fruit. He told the young man he loved to put away his possessions, give them to the poor, and follow him in his new way of life.

In spite of our acquired aversion for the notions of temperance and asceticism in what *Life* magazine's commemorative issue of the 1970's called the "sexed-up, doped-up, hedonistic-heaven of the boom-boom seventies," temperance and its friends are indigenous expressions of the Christian vision of life. We will not be rid of them without throwing overboard the teaching of Jesus himself.

If you were to ask your parents or grandparents why they fasted (if they did) they would probably respond with the language of penance, self-denial, and mortification. They would probably speak of the need for a state of vigilance over our sinful natures that turn so easily from the redeeming grace of Jesus Christ toward self-centeredness. They might say that in the need to control our pleasure urges we must stop short of what is permitted from time to time so that we can build up a proper command over the more unruly parts of our human nature. Though their language might sound foreign to our ears, they are reflecting a valid tradition in Christian practice.

Several months ago I took a few quiet days in the country to do some reading and writing. A constant experience while working on this manuscript was running quite unexpectedly into people who themselves fast. Such was my experience this cloudy spring afternoon. I chatted with one of the neighbors while out for a walk and, in response to a question, told him what I was working on. The man, whose name was Robert, began to describe his own experience, from the perspective that I have just described above.

I fast because our bodies constitute the foundation of our feelings and tendencies. Fasting, by slowing down the drives of the body, helps to control them. Fasting also clears my mind for concentration and makes it easier to pray. I find I can enter more deeply into my own heart when the body is quieted down and the senses are not craving for all sorts of distractions and pleasures.

The experience of talking with him was peaceful because he was peaceful. I went away with the distinct impression that time and the experience of his life were enhancing his own attractiveness as a person. Christian temperance and asceticism is meant to soften and smooth the rough edges of our personalities, to make us more mellow, gentle, and Christlike. Van Kaam and Muto provide the image again:

Rushing waters, harnessed in a reservoir, become a source of energy. Water power is available for constructive purposes. So it is, in a way, with us. These energies need to be channeled if they are to become opportunities for self-emergence in Christ... Lived wisely, discipline has a refining power, a channeling role, a capacity to set me free from the shackles of selfishness and sin.

Any practice of asceticism must always be considered as a means to attain the end of union with God. In the Christian life *per se* there is no value as such in fasting. The value of fasting derives from the interior motivation to aid one's growth in the spiritual life through prudent and gentle correctives to offset the influences of sin in all of its self-centeredness, and to aid one's growth in the positive development of Christ-like virtues. And the *whole person* is the subject of our discipline.

As Father Bob Pelton, a Roman Catholic priest of the Madonna House Community in Combermere, Ontario notes, we are never "finished" because "the deepest fast is the fast from sin, and it is above all the mind and heart that need to be cleansed by surrending the illusory foods they love to feed on."

Fasting has never appealed to me as a way of knowledge or a path to "higher wisdom" or more spiritual awareness, though of course it can be. When I received my first communion after entering the Church at the age of 20, I became aware of how truly hungry I had always been. God revealed to me then how truly Jesus was my *real* food and drink. In my years in the seminary and my early years of priesthood I was not able to remain centered on that hunger and that food, yet I never lost

27

the sense of being, as Flannery O'Connor wrote of one of her strange prophets, "so hungry that I could eat all the loaves and fishes after they were multiplied." When Jesus began to draw me, I knew that he wanted to empty me even further so that he could feed me with himself. I was disgusted with my own mediocrity, but I wasn't sure that I was eager to increase my hunger in order that it might be satisfied! Yet I was sure of two things: that only God and his love could fill my heart and that I wanted Jesus to become more real to me than my own flesh and bones. I saw too that I was useless as a priest as long as I was trying to love with my own love and clinging to a world that had passed away on Calvary.

The deepest fast, of course, is the fast from sin—rebellion, anger, lust, greed, despair, hardness of heart and all the rest—and from egotism, the worship of a life that is in fact death. It is above all the mind and heart that need to be cleansed by surrendering the illusory foods they love to feed on. But fasting from ordinary food is necessary, too; it keeps me honest, mindful of the incarnation and also the resurrection, the Lord's and mine, mindful of my bodiliness and of the aim of purity, which is love. So I don't think about fasting; I just do it, the way I pray and sweep the floor and go to bed. The Lord will use it, has already used it, as he uses everything, to show me the glory of his face within my own heart—and in the hearts of all my sisters and brothers.

Perhaps the heresy of our time is that temperance and asceticism are anti-modern and inhuman, and seemingly deny the goodness of God's creation. This is clouded thinking that confuses a warranted rejection of some of the more "short-circuited" practices of earlier times with a rejection of the very valid foundations of the virtue of temperance and the practice of ascetism.

The universal teaching of the Christian faith, founded on Holy Scripture and the experience of each of us who honestly confronts the selfishness and sin found in ourselves, is that some constant practice of asceticism is a necessary means in order to attain union with God.

2 *If We Don't Know Where We Are We Can't Tell Where We're Going*

> *The end of all our journeying,*
> *is to end up where we began*
> *and to know the place for the first time.*
>
> —T. S. Eliot

Locating the Christian Tradition

A few summers ago, I went with my brother and his wife and a few friends into one of my favorite places in all the world: the Boundary Water Canoe Area of northern Minnesota and the Quetico Provincial Park of Canada. Wilderness canoe camping is a calming, integrating, humbling experience. You never "beat" the wilderness. The most you can ever say is that you survived. There are some seven or eight thousand lakes in this area, a labyrinth of waterways interconnected by rapids, rivers, streams, and overland portage-paths through the woods. If you can't read a topographical map accurately and orient yourself from your map to your surroundings with the help of a compass, you can become hopelessly lost in relatively short order. There are no signs. Anywhere. The nearest ranger's station may be two or three days' paddle away, but even to find *it*, you'd have to know where you are and where it is and be able to stay on track for the distance in between.

On the ninth day of our ten-day trip, we were paddling down Bear Creek, watching for the fork that would take us to Home Lake. In controlled, civil language (now), I can tell you that we were very eager to find that turnoff because every 100 yards or so on this creek there were beaver dams, which means that you have to get out of your canoe, unload all your gear, wetfoot it over the dam, lift and pull the canoe up and over, reload, get in, and start paddling again. After we had negotiated fifteen beaver dams (oh, we counted them, believe me!), the creek began to disappear into tall reeds and marshland.

It was already 3:30 in the afternoon and we'd been on the water since early that morning. We were tired. Our backs ached. And one look around provided all the assurance necessary that this was not, even in wilderness terms, the place to spend a night. The memory that we had planned to make an early camp on a beautiful lake and really enjoy our last evening was vinegar in the wound. We had obviously gone wrong somewhere, but our minds resisted accepting that truth because there was just no way we were prepared psychologically or physically to go back over those beaver dams! We consulted our compasses and pointed grimy fingers at the map saying, "we must be here" or "we must be there."

That day, we all came face to face with a subtle truth: when you don't know where you are, you can't even figure out where to go.

If you *must* know, we did go back over all those beaver dams. We decided that the safest course lay in retracing our steps until we reached a point that we could identify.

And that, I think, is precisely what we need to do with fasting in our spiritual wilderness. We're lost. We need to retrace our steps, to go back to where we've come from. Then, once we have located ourselves in our own Judaeo-Christian environment, once we have our bearings and know what's what, we can move on with a sense of security and sureness about where we're going and where our efforts are taking us.

It's rather sad that Christians who hear about "the three stages of realization" from devotees of Hare Krishna soliciting in airports or who are urged by Zen disciples to strive for enlightenment through meditation cannot speak as knowingly about Christian spirituality. If you did a random interview of people coming out of Christian churches on a Sunday, how many in a hundred do you think would know about the "seven mystical mansions" of St. Teresa of Avila? How many of those interviewed would be able to speak earnestly about the active and passive "dark nights of the soul" described by St. John of the Cross? What percent would be able to be passingly articulate about the "purgative, illuminative and unitive ways" of classical Christian spirituality?

There is a wealth of wisdom in our Christian tradition that we should know about. Our religion should be, above all, *a way of spirituality* that leads to intimate union with God—not just a system of rules and practices. The first believers and followers of the Master Jesus did not call Christianity a "religion," but simply "this new way." Prayer, works of charity, and fasting have traditionally been three pillars on which this "way" of spiritual life was founded.

30

⌈Jesus taught that life in his Kingdom required the right balance among these three basic areas of involvement: doing good to others (almsgiving), intimate relationship to God (prayer), and personal discipline (fasting, as illustrative of the larger area of self-control). The interrelatedness of these three expressions of Christian life cannot be stressed enough.⌋ Part of our brokenness is seen in our inability to maintain them in balance for very long. What has happened to the various Christian churches on the larger scale mirrors what happens to us on the smaller. Certain denominations have become so identified with social action outreach (almsgiving) that it seems to be their whole gospel. Other churches have become known for stressing the importance of the personal, interior, individual response to God (prayer). And still others have been associated in the popular mind with laws governing self-discipline and mortification (symbolized by fasting).

But each is meant to be an aid to the others. *Together* they rightly and harmoniously relate us to God, to others, and to ourselves. It is like the action of a quarterback in passing—there are three distinct movements but all are related: he receives the snap from center, drops back to look for receivers, and throws. No one movement is an absolute; they are all just means to an end.

Or, the interrelatedness of these three movements in Christian life is like the motion of someone answering a doorbell. A lot of front entrances have these little peep-holes in the door. Fasting is like looking through the peep-hole to see who is there (it's a focus of the eye/heart). Prayer is like turning the knob and opening the door (a positive action on our part that invites the presence of the other to come in). And once the guest is within, he has this quiet way of making us sensitive to the needs of others, of telling us to put our jacket on and come back outside with him because down the street he saw somebody who needed help. This is the way prayer and fasting work. If they are genuine responses to the Holy Spirit's urgings in our heart, they will always sensitize us to the needs of others. They will always lead us beyond ourselves, bring us out of our own house and yard and make us more aware of what's going on around us.

So, while the purpose of this book is to focus in a special way upon one of these "movements" in the Christian life—fasting—and to rediscover the riches of our spiritual heritage with regard to this practice, let it be clear at the outset that I have no illusion that fasting, by itself, does all. It is but one pole on a tripod. Stability and balance only come when there is support from every direction. In the past fifteen years, we have been trying to get a focused "picture" of Christian life while relying on a two-legged tripod.

How easily we have shed our traditional fasting practices! The last fifteen years have been like a "molting season," except that there has been no new skin to replace the old one we left behind.

Yes, we've got *diets*—the hard-boiled-egg diet, the grapefruit diet, the brown-rice diet, the Mayo diet, the staple-puncture diet, the Rockefeller diet, the clamped-jaw diet, the drinking-man's diet, the Scarsdale diet, the liquid 900-calories-a-day diet, the HCG 500-calorie-clinic diet, Dr. Stillman's "quick-weight-loss" diet, and Dr. Cott's "ultimate diet"—but these have little to do with *fasting* as a way of spiritual growth. Fasting, as we will be using the term, is an intentional abstention from food and drink on *religious* grounds. The meaning of fasting in this discussion is grasped only if it is seen as an act essentially of the religious spirit.

Fasting and Altered States of Consciousness

It is no accident that fasting has been associated with the human religious response as far back as we can trace it anthropologically. Any fast that goes beyond two or three days generally produces a mild kind of "high," an altered, "higher" state of consciousness. Though we don't often look at religion this way, one of the things religion is about is providing people with an altered state of consciousness.

We, in the Western world, are very suspicious of altered states of consciousness because the only state of consciousness we have baptized as acceptable is what we would call the "ordinary, rational" state of consciousness. Most anything else we have come to associate with drugs, which we associate with abuse, which we label "bad." But, as Andrew Weil notes in his book *The Natural Mind*:

> The desire to alter consciousness periodically is an innate, normal drive analogous to hunger or the sexual drive. Note that I do not say, "desire to alter consciousness by means of chemical agents." Drugs are merely one means of satisfying this drive; there are many others. . . .
>
> The need for periods of nonordinary consciousness is already expressed at ages far too young for it to have much to do with social conditioning; it seems, rather, to be a biological

characteristic of the species. Anyone who watches very young children without revealing his presence will find them regularly practicing techniques that induce striking changes in mental states. Three and four-year-olds, for example, commonly whirl themselves into vertiginous stupors. They hyperventilate and have other children squeeze them around the chest until they faint. They also choke each other to produce loss of consciousness. . . . It is most interesting that children quickly learn to keep this sort of play out of sight of grownups, who instinctively try to stop them. . . . Children learn very quickly that they must pursue antisocial behavior patterns if they wish to continue to alter consciousness regularly. Hence the secret meetings in cloakrooms, garages, and playground corners where they can continue to whirl, choke each other, and perhaps, sniff cleaning fluids or gasoline.

We seem, in other words, to be born with a drive to experience episodes of altered consciousness. This drive expresses itself at very early ages in all children in activities designed to cause disturbance of ordinary awareness. To an adult observer these practices seem perverse and dangerous, but in most cases adults have simply forgotten their own identical experiences as children.

Before we can even mention, without raising anxieties, that fasting does set into motion in the body certain chemical changes that can result in a mild, altered state of consciousness, it is necessary to balance our usually negative notion of altered consciousness. Altered from what? From ordinary waking consciousness, which is "normal" only in the strict sense of "statistically most frequent." "Normal" here has no connotation of "good," "worthwhile," or "healthy." Various altered states of consciousness that are not "normal waking consciousness" but which could be considered "good," "worthwhile," or "healthy" for us nonetheless (given the proper circumstances) are: sleep, daydreaming, trance, meditation, hypnosis, general anesthesia, mystic rapture, and various chemical "highs" induced for socially acceptable purposes.

It is noteworthy that most of the world's highest religious and philosophic thought originated in altered states of consciousness in individuals like Gautama, St. Paul, and Mohammed. It is also relevant to note that creative genius has long been correlated with psychosis (another "unordinary" state) and that intuitive genius is often associated with daydreaming, meditation, and other nonordinary modes of consciousness.

It can be soberly said, therefore, that altered states of consciousness have great potential for strongly positive psychic development. They appear to be the ways to more effective and fuller use of the nervous system, to development of creative and intellectual faculties, and to attainment of certain kinds of thought that have been deemed exalted by all who have experienced them.

From time to time, we need to alter our state of consciousness, and it has been one of the functions of religion to help us do this. Lighting, sound, and smell are effective means for altering consciousness. Consider how religion has used candles, music, and incense in its rituals. Consider, too, how many people have protested when, in its recent liturgical reforms, the Roman Catholic Church cut back on much of its pomp and pageantry, its "smells and bells." "It isn't the same anymore" was an oft-heard comment. People seemed to be trying to convey that the "stripped-down" liturgy didn't take them out of themselves, didn't make them feel awe and mystery, didn't alter their ordinary state of consciousness and graft them into another Reality present to them. The new rites feel, perhaps, too "ordinary."

There may well be a strong correlation between this and the fact that Eastern religious sects have attracted many lapsed Christians in the last two decades. The Eastern ways, with their emphasis upon mystery, subjective and higher states of consciousness, are fulfilling a need. Through meditation, fasting, chanting, etc., they are providing spiritually hungry people with a methodology for achieving an altered, higher state of consciousness.

When the North American Indians sent a brave off into the wilderness on a fast, it was a holy quest for guidance from the Great Spirit. The fast was intended to help "bring on the vision." It is this dimension of fasting, seen as an act essentially of the religious spirit, that it is our purpose to recover.

Fasting and Primitive Religion

Fasting has been closely linked with humankind's intimate sense of religion in almost all times and places. Some would dismiss the manifestations it has taken in primitive cultures as "magical." To be sure, it has taken magical expressions, but even these related to man's sense of a Transcendent Being particular to that culture and society. What is significant is that beneath the use of fasting was a desire and intention to contact the gods.

The faster in a primitive society whose motive was what we would call "magical" attempted to gain ascendancy over nature by using the fast as a hold over its powers. This wasn't all that much different from the way the Hebrews used fasting later—to bend the ear of God toward them in mercy and favor. In primitive religions in which natural occurrences or objects of nature were considered to influence events, a fast in honor of, for example, the lord of the storm, was invoked. Also, demons were commonly thought to enter the body of a person through food; the ritual of fasting was then necessary for the individual who wanted to communicate with God. One became a "pure vessel" of the spirit of the Transcendent by exorcising the demons through fasting.

In other times and places, fasting has been viewed as an "ethical" expression. The person who fasts from ethical motivation seeks either to strengthen his own moral fiber or, transcending himself, that of the community. An outstanding example of one who fasted not for personal but for community benefit was Mahatma Gandhi whose fasts were undertaken primarily in atonement for the violent excesses of those who opposed the British government in India (his own opposition was nonviolent). The spirit of Gandhi pricks the soul of our generation, and stirs up our long-buried religious intuitions. We are in the process of going through our attic and recapitulating and re-experiencing the wisdom of our human family's past.

We do not know where to go or what to do until we know where we are on the map of Judaeo-Christian history. Failure to locate ourselves in terms of where we've come jeopardizes the rest of our journey. It would be easy to go around in circles, not benefiting from the explorations and chartings of those who have gone before us.

There has been a tremendous amount of exploring and testing already done in the quest for human fulfillment. What is it that compels us to leave the logbooks of our ancestral pilgrims closed, to believe that the information contained there doesn't apply to the human situation today?

We have succeeded in organizing and cataloging this information better than ever before, but have we *learned* everything from it? Why was something in me surprised recently when I asked a priest whom I respected what were his few favorite books? "The writings of the Desert Fathers and other early Fathers of the Church," he said. "Why those?" I pursued, somewhat caught by surprise that it wasn't a book written within the past ten years. "Because," he said, "I think the Holy Spirit was communicating some very essential teachings to those early Christian communities about what it means to genuinely follow 'the way' of Jesus." His response forced me to confront within myself the reaction that "if it hasn't been written recently, it won't be in touch with the needs of our times." There are, however, certain fundamentals of human experience. Earlier writings are often the freshest on these basic values; more contemporary writings are a rephrasing of the original insights into language more palatable to modern ears.

If someone were to take a sampling of our "culture" today through newspapers, magazines, television, theater, advertising and try to distill from it a sense of where our values are, what would emerge as *our* "way to fulfillment?"

In our society we simply do not encounter all that much genuine fulfillment. I have an acquaintance who could fairly be set forth as a paradigm of the consumer society: a dazzling variety of magazines lie scattered about his room. His wardrobe would make the editors of *Gentleman's Quarterly* smile approvingly. The areas of the globe that he has not personally visited are diminishing rapidly, and there is not a conversational subject that you could introduce in which you would not find him a stimulating partner of discourse. But I experience in him a restlessness, an insecurity, a constant reaching for the next new fashion-fad or hit play. Our unlimited freedoms and resources have not brought us unlimited fulfillment. The time has come for the consumer society to, in the words of Edward Farrell, generate its antithesis, "the man who stands against the conditioned reflex, the man who is free not to consume, the man who can fast."

The person who fasts stands in a noble tradition. In the religious experience of humankind, fasting has always been a prelude and means to a deeper spiritual life. Failure to control the amount we eat and drink disturbs the inner order of our body-spirit. Fasting is a choice to regulate our eating or to abstain from food at certain times in order to put our attention on something more important to us than ourselves or our sensory appetites. How far back does this practice go in our Judaeo-Christian history?

Fasting in Old Testament Times

The Hebrews, the Aramaeans, the Arabs, and the Ethiopians all used the same word for it, a word that appears in both early and late Old Testament writings: *tsoum*. The word in its first level of meaning signifies "withholding all natural food from the body," especially for a religious purpose. The second level of meaning included an expression of sorrow for sins and a penitential offering. Together

36

they convey the idea of voluntary deprivation of the bodily appetites for the purpose of orienting the human spirit to Someone greater. The act of fasting was undertaken to create an inner awareness of one's creatureliness, interior poverty, and alienation from the AllHoly.

There appear to have been three occasions for fasting among the Hebrews. *First, as a preparation for some religious duty.* Thus Moses remained fasting on Sinai for forty days and nights when about to receive the Commandments (Exodus 34:28), and Daniel fasted for a considerable time seeking to know God's will (Daniel 3-10:2). *Secondly, as an accompaniment or manifestation of mourning.* David, for example, mourned Saul with fasting (I Samuel 31:13, II Samuel 1:12). The fact that David did *not* fast after the death of the child he had fathered by Bathsheba caused surprise in his attendants, which suggests that the usual procedure was to fast after a death. And *thirdly*, the Hebrews fasted *as an act of humility and atonement* to conciliate Yahweh. Illustrations of this are numerous: Ahab fasted to avert the disaster predicted by Elijah (I Kings 21:27-29); Nehemiah fasted over the sad condition of Jerusalem (Nehemiah 1:4); and the whole people fasted in times of peril and misfortune (II Chronicles 20:3; Jeremiah 36:9; I Maccabees 3:47).

The Mosaic Law obliged the people to observe only one day of fasting in the year: the Day of Atonement, or the Feast of Expiations. On that day, the tenth day of the seventh month (Kippur), the high priest sent a scapegoat out into the desert, symbolically laden with the sins of the people who, meanwhile, were fasting in prayer that Yahweh would take from his sight their sins as individuals and as a nation. This day of fasting was taken very seriously—anyone who decided to satisfy his other hunger pains on this day was thrown out of the community.

In post-exilic times, the days on which disasters had occurred were commemorated as fast days. For example, four regular fasts were added to commemorate the four main events connected with the destruction of Jerusalem and the exile (Zechariah 8:19), but these had only a light obligation. Certain rituals accompanied the fast, like the rending of clothing and the placing of ashes on the head. Fasting seems to have been the supplication best suited to obtain God's mercy: when the people came to the point of giving up their food and drink, they were sending God a message that they meant business this time.

Whereas the women of our time have been known to lay out an elegant meal to get to the heart of their beloved, we see Esther,

Judith, Sara, and the daughter of Raguel employing a reverse tactic: they *fast* to move God to grant them a desired favor. There is something vitally personal about this: certainly a "God of the Philosophers" would not be swayed by such wile and pressure. An "Unmoved Mover" would itself be swayed by such wile and pressure.

An "Unmoved Mover" would itself be likely to remain unmoved; a "First Cause" would surely be unaffected by such despicably emotional behavior. But the God of the Israelites—now that's another story! Here is One who suffers fits of jealousy, who succumbs to possessiveness, who is enraged when the eyes of his betrothed begin to stray and linger upon the "competition." It is not surprising that one would expect *this* God to be moved and affected when his people sought his attention in a deeply real and no nonsense manner. The Israelites' use of fasting reveals to us something terribly poignant and profound about their relationship with God: it was incredibly *personal*. No sense of remoteness here. No sense of a God who winds up the world like a clock and walks off to leave it ticking on its own. No way. They don't fast to an abstraction. They fast because they want it to have an impact. They want it to be heard. They *expect* results. And they got them!

* * *

There is an important characteristic of fasting in the Hebrew world that we must not miss. For them, fasting was not just a body-thing or a soul-thing. For the Hebrews there was just one entity: the enfleshed spirit, the animated body, the soul incarnated. A unified embodied-spirit.

On the hillside of the campus where I went to college, there are five big letters set into the earth in whitewashed stone: DMACT. They stand for five Latin words that were the motto of St. John Bosco, founder of the Salesian Fathers and Brothers who run the college: "*Da Mihi Animas, Coetera Tolle*" (Give me souls, take away the rest). The Hebrews wouldn't have understood that motto. Why, they would have wanted to know, do you either separate the bodysoul into two distinct realities, or call the animated body just a "soul"? For them, the human person was an indivisible unity. Nothing demonstrates their sense of this unity better than their practice of fasting: the interior sorrow and conversion of the heart ("spirit") were expressed through the physical fast of abstaining from corporal nourishment.

When the prophets verbally lashed out at those fasts that were filled with exterior ritual (e.g., Isaiah 58:3-11, Joel 2:12-13) but lacked the inner conversion of the heart, they did not intend at all that people just stop their physical fasting altogether. They were basically saying that a clock without the inner workings doesn't do what a clock is supposed to do. They were attacking our natural tendency to go through the motions and feel very smug and selfsatisfied and secure because we're "keeping the law." But a new bicycle without any air in the tires isn't going to make any little child jump up and down. And neither will the religious practice of fasting be pleasing to God if there's no "heart" in it. And so the prophets said: Put it to rest. There's nothing of life and growth in it. It's just an empty form.

In Isaiah 58, there's a dialogue between the people and God in which God lays it right on the line:

People:
Why do we fast, and you do not see it?
Afflict ourselves, and you take no note of it?

God:
Lo, on your fast day you carry out your own
    pursuits, and drive all your laborers.
Yes, your fast ends in quarreling and
    fighting, striking with wicked claw.
Would that today you might fast
    so as to make your voices heard on high!
Is this the manner of fasting I wish;
    of keeping a day of penance:
That a man bow his head like a reed,
    and lie in sackcloth and ashes?
Do you call this a fast,
    a day acceptable to the Lord?

And then God goes on to stress the importance of the harmonious balance between fasting, doing good to others, and intimacy with God:

This, rather, is the fasting that I wish:
    releasing those bound unjustly,

39

untying the thongs of the yoke,
Setting free the oppressed,
   breaking every yoke;
Sharing your bread with the hungry,
   sheltering the oppressed and the homeless;
Clothing the naked when you see them,
   and not turning your back on your own.

In the Old Testament, fasting is a total experience. The person stands before God as an enfleshed spirit, owning his littleness, recognizing her dependency, begging for forgiveness. To fast is to adopt the conduct and deportment that becomes a marvelous but flawed creature who can't seem to keep the boat on a straight rudder for very long before a corrective touch needs to be applied to the wheel to keep the bow on course. In all cases, fasting is to be accompanied by an interior surrender of self to God. It's an action that says: "You're the greatest. You mean more to me than life itself, which is what the food I set aside symbolizes for me."

Old Testament fasting appears to be an act of self-renunciation and self-discipline that is designed to make an impression on God. Voluntarily going without nourishment or anything else agreeable to the senses seemed to be the ideal means of expressing one's dependence upon God. A meal is meant to be an occasion and expression of joy, so going without it expressed mourning, a desire for healing or spiritual guidance. Abstention from food was an appeal for divine mercy, for the all-important change of heart, and for forgiveness. It manifested penitence and the will for atonement.

The Teaching of Jesus on Fasting

When Jesus arrived, the practice of fasting, as we have just seen it, was in vogue in Israel: the Jews fasted on Mondays and Thursdays. It's more than just "interesting" to see what Jesus' perspective is on fasting, because the Christian finds in Jesus what God is like, and what God thinks, the Christian learns from Jesus. So—does Jesus have anything new to add?

He does.

Joy.

Joy, he says: it's got to be joyful.

40

When Jesus began to teach his disciples about fasting, he did not oppose the practice that he found prevalent in Israel. He just said that those who went through all the external motions, without ever having it touch their hearts, were a bunch of phonies. In this he is entirely consistent with the teaching embodied in the dialogue between God and the people which we just read from the Book of Isaiah. There is never a question for him as to whether his followers *should* fast; he deals more with the "how" and "when." His first statement about fasting was along the lines of "*how not to*":

> When you fast, you are not to look glum as the hypocrites do. They change the appearance of their faces so that others may see they are fasting. I assure you, they are already repaid. When you fast, see to it that you comb your hair and wash your face. In that way no one can see you are fasting but your Father who is hidden; and your Father who sees what is hidden will repay you (Matthew 6:16-18).

Beyond this kind of statement, the disciples are not able to pin him down to any new specific regulations on the nature and frequency of fasting. He prefers to talk about attitudes and essential meanings. Fasting, the way he sees it, is a sign and symbol of the conversion to God that takes place in the heart. That is to say, secretly. So there's something out of kilter when I tell my secretary or co-worker, loud enough for everyone in the office to hear, "no food for me today—I'm fasting." The conversion to the Father has the intimacy of little secrets between nuptial partners and, therefore, fasting from now on has to be in secret.

That's not all. Fasting before God, the Father who receives mercifully all those who turn to him, is JOY. There is no room for melancholy signs of mourning. This new accent of joy in fasting is highlighted in Jesus' second statement on the subject in the Gospel of Matthew. The occasion for it was the shock and scandal of John the Baptist's disciples over the fact that Jesus and his followers did not fast as they and the Pharisees did. It must have been an intriguing encounter, kind of like Ford going to General Motors and saying "Why aren't you building your cars with four wheels anymore?"

Jesus replied:

> How can the wedding guests go in mourning so long as the groom is with them? When the day comes that the groom is taken away, then they will fast (9:15).

It's a great rejoinder, and there is so much more there than we usually find in two sentences worth of words. The way in which the reign of God is rushing into the world through the presence and ministry of Jesus leaves only room right now for joy and thanksgiving. Jesus has come as the Bridegroom to establish a mystical marriage with God's people. "The bridegroom is the one to whom the bride belongs; the bridegroom's friend stands by and listens, and he is glad when he hears the bridegroom's voice" (John 3:29).

Before the crucifixion it was a time of celebrating the nuptial promises, a time for announcing the "good news": the Kingdom of Heaven is close at hand—indeed, it is already in your midst. The joyous exterior when a Christian fasts has a profound meaning that is basic to the Christian faith: Jesus is bringing new wine, a total transformation is happening. Henceforth, the sign of Christian fasting is to be joy and charity. Fasting is no longer just the self-renunciation and self-discipline arduously forged by the human will and designed to make an impression on God. Fasting is now a recognition of something new that is already set in motion, though not yet completed: the reign of God in our midst. When this is grasped, that the reign of God is HERE, fasting is a reflex response, an aftermath.

The joy that animates Christian fasting is like the joy of someone who has been told by relatives that he or she has been handsomely included in their will and, as a matter of fact, they can start drawing upon their inheritance anytime there is need since it's going to be all theirs someday anyway. The joy that marks Christian fasting is the kind of joy felt by a couple who have not been able to have their own natural children at the time they are told that their name is approaching the top of the adoption list and soon their hopes will be realized. The joy that pervades Christian fasting is like the joy a young actor, singer, or dancer experiences when receiving a first part and realizing that the breakthrough has arrived and there's so much possibility ahead. The joy that characterizes Christian fasting is like the joy a person feels when she has just got a new car (even though only the down payment has been made) and vacation is just around the corner.

"But the time will come when the groom is taken away. Then, they will fast." After Jesus gave his life for his Bride, his people, his friends, there is a period of waiting for his second and final coming. And during this time, his faithful are not idle, but wait with busy hands, in vigilant preparation for his return. Fasting is part of this future-oriented waiting until the Bridegroom comes in all his splendor and glory.

The Old Testament spirit of fasting was surpassed in the sense that fasting now points for the Christian toward participation in the death and resurrection of the Lord, Jesus. It is now marked by a spirit of joyful expectation and striving toward his return.

Does this mean that it won't "hurt" anymore, that it will now be easy to fast? No, there's still a "bite" to it. Our stomachs will still growl and we may even get a bit of a headache and it's unlikely that our breath will pass for perfume. But that's as it should be, because while the work of God's reign in our hearts *is* at large among us, it is not yet completed. Or, as one of my friends is fond of saying: "It's already Christmas, not yet Easter" (referring generally to our feeling that there is still more to come). Perhaps it would be more theologically accurate to say: "It's already Easter, not yet the Parousia" (a fluid, musical Greek word referring to the Lord's coming in glory).

In other words, our hearts still need softening, we still have difficulty making God the still point at the center of our frenetic distracted lives. And thus we continue to have need of those practices and disciplines that help us readjust our priorities and remind us where our real treasure lies. We all find in our lives pockets of pride, selfishness, a will to control other's lives, a tendency to give ourselves over to sensory pleasures. The example of Jesus himself going into the desert for forty days tells us that there will be little control or moderation in our personal lives unless there is also something of dying—dying to those areas of our lives where we *too* alive. For example, our egotism and self-concern can block our discernment of what God is asking of us, can cause us to resist conforming ourselves to the will of the Father because of what it will cost us. Jesus prepared himself by fasting for what lay ahead of him, and his example instructs us at least as much as his words. It is in the spirit, with his eyes on lasting treasure, that St. Paul wrote:

All the athletes at the games go into strict training: they do this just to win a wreath that will wither away, but we do it for a wreath that will never wither (I Corinthians 9:25).

3   *After Jesus: Christian Fasting*

> *Almost everywhere and at all times*
> *fasting has held a place of great*
> *importance since it is closely linked*
> *with the intimate sense of religion.*
> *Perhaps this is the explanation for*
> *the demise of fasting in our day.*
> *When the sense of God diminishes,*
> *fasting disappears. Perhaps more*
> *accurately, when the vision fades,*
> *i.e., when the wisdom, language and*
> *tradition are no longer understood,*
> *the habit and practice wither away.*
>
> —Edward Farrell

At bottom, I am a frustrated craftsman. I can wander for hours in an artisans' exposition, admiring woven fabrics, discussing batiking methods, running my fingers over wood that has been worked by human hands, and thrilling to the graceful flow of earthtone pottery. When I was in graduate school in Washington, D.C., my favorite late-night haunt was "The Potter's House." To be sure, I liked the hot mulled cider that warmed my hands as I cradled the rustic mug, leisurely sipping, but in the main I liked the place because it was about as close as I could come, in that setting, to a cherished fantasy in which I sit at a potter's wheel in my simple cabin in the woods with moist clay oozing between my fingers.

Once I actually did get to sit at a potter's wheel. Five of us were running an inner-city summer program in San Francisco and the team member in charge of arts and crafts had obtained a potter's wheel. I remember the instructions well, for this was no casual experience.

First of all, I had to choose the clay that would have the proper plasticity and texture for the vessel I wanted to shape. I then kneaded the moist clay until all the air bubbles had been forced out of it, and centered the ball of clay on the potter's wheel. Not only the ball of clay had to be centered, but I had to be centered, completely in balance with the wheel. Then I began to shape the vessel, molding the mass of clay into a cylinder by gently drawing it upward, slowly pushing on the outside while shaping from the inside. As the potter's wheel made its revolutions, my fingers shaped the vessel from the inside, making it swell at the base and narrow at the neck. This "inside work" is possible only because of the presence of the potter's steadying hand on the outside, gently working in tandem with the pressure of his fingers from the inside. Throughout the whole process, both the clay and one's fingers must remain moist lest the fingers catch on to the clay and destroy the fragile shape of the vessel that begins to emerge.

As I have studied theology and accumulated more experience in the spiritual life,* I have returned periodically to my experience at the potter's wheel as a good image for the kind of shaping or being shaped that the spiritual life requires. We select a few practices that will give our lives the proper malleability they will need to remain in line with the design of our vocation. Then the gentle kneading, molding and being drawn into the chosen vessel may begin. The slow, gradual push and pull of our spirituality shapes our lives from the inside as we try to cooperate with and be responsive to the fingers of the Master Potter who wishes to mold us into a vessel of integral proportion and refined beauty.

The exercises of prayer, fasting, and good works are like the caring push and pull to direct our lives into a deeper intimacy with God. They represent "keeping our clay moist."

It is not thou that shapest God;
it is God that shapest thee.
If then thou art the work of God,
await the hand of the Artist
who does all things in due season.
Offer him thy heart soft and tractable

---

*I have a strong dislike for the term "spiritual life" because it dichotomizes our religious experience from the flesh-and-blood world. I do not have a "spirit" life and a "body" life. I just have *my* life, the life of an embodied spirit. It is the whole of me that is to find delight in the Lord, not just my "spirit."

and keep the form in which the Artist
has fashioned thee. Let thy clay be moist,
lest thou grow hard and lose the imprint
of his fingers.

—St. Iranaeus

Certain conditions foster nearness to God, such as silence, fidelity to prayer, recollection, and ascetical practices. Yet, no amount of desire, willing or manipulating can do more than prepare us for the gift of the awareness of his presence. We often use the phrase that we want to be "closer to God," but ultimately what that phrase really means is "becoming aware of God," for we are already close to him. As a Christmas card I received so beautifully phrased it: Our hearts are his birthplace, our lives are his home. "He is not really far from any of us," St. Paul writes, "since it is in him that we live and move and exist." It is we who are seldom "at home," seldom in touch with the deepest and most fundamental reality of our lives. Becoming a more spiritual or religious person means becoming aware of our rootedness in God, of our dependence on him for every breath we take, every thought we have.

Following the Spirit's Lead

"What are we," the Psalmist asks, "that you have made us little less than the angels?" One of life's great challenges to us is to accept the fact that we are from a divine Source, that we—each of us—are unique and irreplaceable, the art work of God. And a second of life's great tasks is for us to integrate with this first truth another: that this unspeakably complex, free, enfleshed spirit which we are, has become, by our own choices, crippled. The Holy Spirit opens our eyes and gives us the humility to recognize as we grow in the "spiritual" life just how wounded our human nature is. It may have been God's design for us that we hold all our basic desires and appetites in perfect and harmonious balance, but at this point in our history we must honestly admit that we are not capable of pulling that nifty little tightrope act off by ourselves.

We need the Spirit of God. The farther reaches of our human nature under grace (which is simply God's gift of his Spirit to our hearts) is still limitless, even reaching for divinity itself. But it is only

46

by the Spirit of Jesus Christ, who himself, freed from all sin and unruly concupiscences, fasted "violently" for forty days, that we will learn how to fast in a truly Christian way. The Holy Spirit not only gives fasting its true significance, but is absolutely necessary to animate the fast so that it goes beyond mere technique. Only the Holy Spirit can connect our fasting with changing our hearts, with opening them more fully to the Father. Our efforts on the corporal and psychological levels by way of technique, will-power, desires and the like *dispose* us and play a very important role, but without the current of God's Spirit flowing through them it would be like turning on a TV set that is not plugged in. We are, of course, talking here about fasting for a very particular kind of reason—the "reason" of a creature's relationship to its Creator.

There are reasons why people fast that don't *necessarily* relate in any conscious, explicit way to our sense of relationship to God:

    To lose weight the quickest and easiest way
    To feel better physically and mentally
    To look and feel younger
    To save money
    To give the whole system a rest
    To clean out the body
    To lower blood-pressure and cholesterol levels
    To cut down on smoking and drinking
    To get more out of sex
    To let the body heal itself
    To relieve tension
    To end dependence on drugs
    To sleep better
    To digest food better
    To regulate bowels
    To feel euphoric
    To sharpen the senses
    To quicken mental processes
    To save time
    To boost self-esteem
    To learn better eating habits
    To share with the hungry
    To gain control of oneself
    To call attention to social issues
    To slow the aging process

47

As good and worthwhile and healthy and whatever else all those things might be, we are yet looking for something *more* in fasting: that it be an act of *religion*. Religion, in its root meaning (*re-ligare*) means to re-tie, to re-connect us to God, to bind us again to the Source from whom we came and to whom we are on pilgrimage. Only the Spirit of God can enable the act of fasting to do that for us. In and of itself, like any other external human act, it is ambivalent. In and of itself, as the list above demonstrates, it is religiously an indifferent act. It can even be spiritually *dangerous* in that it can become an achievement of human virtue, a trophy on our mental shelf, a source of spiritual pride. It happened to the Pharisees who were "professionally religious" and it can certainly happen to us. Since the particular purpose of this book is to rediscover fasting precisely as a *religious* act, it must be declared clearly and unambiguously that the worth of fasting as a religious act lies in the faith and love of which it is the expression. Without such faith and love its meaning lies somewhere else.

The hinge-pin that makes fasting one thing or the other is my *intention*, which is the doorway for the Spirit. If I am open and inviting and willing it, the Spirit can make of my fast a powerful symbol of my own awareness of my creatureliness before my Creator-God; the Spirit can make of my physical hunger a symbol of my soul's deepest hungerings; the Spirit can give me an experience of God's goodness and compassion and stir up within me a deep sense of repentance and desire to change my life; the Spirit can reveal to me the fragmentation of my existence and push me, through fasting, towards true life, where

> All I want is to know Christ
> and the life flowing from his resurrection;
> likewise to know how to share in his sufferings,
> being formed into the pattern of his death (Philippians 3:10).

What is new in the world after Jesus? His teachings, his example, and most of all, his gift to us, the Holy Spirit, who makes it possible for us to live both. "And since we live by the Spirit, let us follow the Spirit's lead" (Galatians 5:25). If we fast following the Spirit's lead, the Spirit will bring forth in us, through fasting, her fruit.

> Let me put it like this: if you
> are guided by the Spirit you will

48

be in no danger of yielding to
self-indulgence, since self-indulgence
is the opposite of the Spirit;
the Spirit is totally against such
a thing . . . (Galatians 5:16).

Do we want to fast in the Spirit of Jesus? And when we try, how do we know that we are? The best test is always this: we will know that our fasting is under her guidance by the fruit produced.

The fruit of the Spirit is—

love
joy
peace
patient endurance
kindness
generosity
faith
mildness
and chastity (Galatians 5:22).

Fasting in the Early Christian Church

Following the example of Christ and the apostles, the early Christians practiced fasting. The primitive Church took over the custom of fasting from Judaism, from which comes the oldest injunction we have concerning Christian fasting, i.e., two days per week were designated as fast days. The Jews had observed Monday and Thursday, and whoever wished to fast did so on those two days, though there was no general command to fast. The Gentile-Christian churches appointed Wednesday and Friday, demonstrating a dependence upon Judaism by the designation of two days but evidencing a protest to Judaism by the change of days from Monday and Thursday to Wednesday and Friday.

As we have seen, Jesus established no specific legislation on fasting, but left it to the church to determine, underlining the critical importance of investing the practice with certain attitudes. During the time of his letters to the young Christian churches (thirty to fifty years after Jesus' death and resurrection), St. Paul taught the necessity of fasting and used his own example to encourage others. In his reference to "frequent fastings" (II Corinthians 11:27; 6:5) we have an indication not merely of involuntary periods of hunger but of a Pauline practice that he wished to be imitated by other Christians. It's not too hard to understand why Paul would not be inclined to legislate too precisely in this matter: one of his heaviest themes is that we are not saved by our observance of any static and uniform laws. For Paul the key concept is freedom and liberty in the Spirit. We must first of all grasp the profound and too-good-to-believe reality that we have been *given, freely*, as a *gift*, the divine life-giving Spirit of God who dwells within us. Once that life-changing realization has penetrated our thick heads and seeped through to our crusty hearts, there will be an implosion of gratitude that will find us doing things like fasting and praying and treating others kindly because we are just so full of thanks that we have an utter need to express it somehow. And we will do all those things with an inner quiet joy and peace and serenity. None will have to force us, no matter what they do to us, because nothing, *nothing* else matters quite so much as this: to be loved so completely, so passionately, so unconditionally. And to respond to it.

We find in the early Christian community the "Big Three" of prayer, fasting, and doing good to others. They move in such beautiful harmony with one another, like three interlocked wheels of a watch, whose smooth functioning-in-tandem is necessary for the instrument to do its work. Before Paul and Barnabas set off on a special mission to bring the good news of Jesus Christ to others, the prophets and teachers and whole community fasted and prayed, and "after they had fasted and prayed, they imposed hands on them and sent them off" (Acts 13:2-3; 14:23). Note here the three "wheels" are all interlocked.

The early Christian writers—Justin, Polycarp, Hermas, Pseudo-Barnabas—constantly exhorted their readers to fast. There are a number of books like the *Didache*, the *Canons of the Apostolic Didascalias*, and the *Apostolic Constitutions* that are very important because they give us a record of what was going on among the earliest Christian communities. In the *Didache*, which is one of the most ancient documents of nonscriptural literature, written before the ruin of Jerusalem in A.D. 70, we learn that fasts were prescribed for Wednesdays and Fridays. And it is interesting to note in this document, too, that a line in Matthew's Gospel ("Pray for your persecutors") appears with an alteration performed upon it: "Fast for your persecutors." Something like that tells us that they grasped very well that fasting is a matter of the heart—and not only good for changing *your own* heart, but that of your enemy as well!

We pick up a couple of other things from the *Didache*, too. In preparing for a baptism, both the baptizer and the candidate fasted. (I wonder how that would go over with baptizers today!) The Lord's Supper was to be received fasting as well. Out of such practices, the fast before Easter developed (Easter being the time when the new members were received into the eucharistic community through baptism). Easter is the only annual festival of the Church going back to the first century, and the gradual appointment of a general fast beforehand was only to observe a custom that was everywhere considered a matter of course anyway. The first clear evidence of this custom turns up in the second century, where we find the day before Easter as a fast day in one place, the two or more days before Easter in another place, and the custom of fasting for forty hours before the Easter celebration in yet another place. In general, the idea was to make the duration of the fast coextensive with the amount of time Christ spent in the tomb. Another ancient tome, the Syriac *Didascalia*, tells us that on the night before Easter the faithful assembled in the church and the fasting ceased at the liturgical ritual at which they celebrated the resurrection of the Lord.

In the course of the third century the fast was extended to the six days of Holy Week; the innovation was combined with the ancient custom (of fasting a day or two before Easter) by making the fast on the last two days more strict. Fasting was based in principle upon the suffering of Christ. The commemoration of the death of Jesus on Friday is very old, and it is possible that, from the beginning, the death of Jesus was commemorated every Friday, just as his resurrection was celebrated every Sunday.

Another third-century development in Rome was the establishment of a *third* (in addition to Wednesday and Friday) weekly fast day: Saturday. It seems that the Saturday fast was considered a weekly repetition of the fast before Easter. This Roman innovation, however, did not spread widely. The East always declined to adopt it, and when in the West three fast days per week appeared too many, it was Wednesday, not Saturday, that was given up.

At the beginning of the fourth century, in the time of a great persecution of Christians, the forty-day fast was introduced on the analogy of the forty-day fast of Jesus in the desert, and Lent was born. The custom of different churches varied in the fourth century, but by the fifth a certain amount of harmony was reached by fixing the fast either at six or at seven weeks. Rome observed six, and this is the present custom of the Latin Church.

If you're duly impressed already with the people's zeal for fasting, we're only halfway there! From the middle of the fourth century, the birth of Jesus was celebrated on December 25, and it struck the people as natural that, like Easter, the new high festival should also be preceded by a forty-day fast! Rome, a moderating influence even then, reduced the original time to the present four weeks of Advent.

Just how seriously did the people take all these fasting days? Well, the requirement of fasting during the whole of Lent and Advent proved too difficult even for the segment of the population that hardly knew any regular times for meals and was accustomed to only meager and primitive food. Already in the fourth century, during the lifetime of people who had themselves witnessed the implementation of these customs, it seemed to emerge by consensus that they would fast two or three weeks but not the whole forty days. Fasting, for them, by the way, was generally understood as abstinence of all food until evening, or one meal a day, which was to be as simple as possible. In the first century, that translated into bread, salt, and water. Later on, fruits and eggs, sometimes fish and even poultry were allowed, so that the fasting was finally limited to the prohibition of flesh-meat and wine. To limit thus the enjoyment of food to the barest necessities, or to refrain from certain designated articles of food, constituted "abstinence" in the technical sense.

The increasing effort to structure the fasting experience within this or that fixed time, and to make distinctions between fasting and abstinence, introduces the danger of approaching the practice in a legalistic way. As we have noted earlier, the problem with ascetical practices has always been the difficulty of keeping the means from becoming ends in themselves.

The Influence of Early Monasticism

The "means-and-end mix-up" has a long history, traceable to the influence of pagan cultures and philosophies that were contemporaneous with the early stages of Christianity's growth. The early church was not able to keep the strands of Platonism,

Manichaeism, and Stoicism out of its garment. The place where we see some of this flawed fabric being handed on is in early monasticism whose origins and first developments came from the fourth century. It was out of monasticism that many popular practices grew and were adopted by the people.

As long as the threat of persecution by the Roman Emperor remained, martyrdom (which was seen as the highest grace that could come to anyone) was normally held to be the final stage in the spiritual ascent of a Christian seeking perfection. When peace came to the church, Christianity was welcomed in the world and installed itself very comfortably there. The flood of often superficial or selfish conversions both in the masses and among the elite was bound to bring about a relaxation of spiritual tension within the church.

In these conditions it is understandable that flight from the world appeared to be the most favorable if not the necessary condition for attaining holiness. There was, in fact, a creeping sanctification of withdrawal: any denial of the Christians' relationship to the material world somehow made the person holier.

Christian monasticism turned to its own use the deeply rooted ideals whose equivalent are found in the varied civilizations of India, Central Asia, China, and pre-Columban America: solitude, asceticism and contemplation. In contrast to the pride of newly converted intellectuals who brought to Christianity the aristocratic traditions of their pagan masters, monasticism reaffirmed, as Franciscanism was later to do in the thirteenth century, the preeminence of simple people, which is one of the essential aspects of the Gospel message.

The life of St. Anthony, the "father of monks" who died in 356, demonstrates the style of early monasticism. He broke all his ties with the world and gave himself up to a solitary life. His long career can be divided into three stages, each of which was a search for more complete isolation. The challenge was always, one way or another, to master the passions completely, and thereby to attain tranquillity.

Christian asceticism, however, is not an end in itself. Its purpose is to prepare and orient the whole personality for mystical experience. It is a means to that end.

From our own experience it should not surprise us that the means and the end sometimes become confused, as was the case with some of the first Egyptian monks, rough Coptic peasants, who were used to so low a standard of living that their eagerness to repress concupiscence often led them to disconcerting excesses in such matters as privation of food and sleep. It was in this context that fasting often became an end in itself, separate from the path of mystical relationship with God.

Paradoxically, or rather by a strange reversal of roles, these hermits attracted crowds of visitors who came to ask for their prayers, their advice, or simply for a good example. Some of the visitors, edified and comforted, returned to their daily routine. Others, deeply affected by the example of the ascetics, installed themselves beside them, placed themselves under their direction, and tried to imitate their way of life.

Even during the lifetime of St. Anthony, monasticism spread throughout the whole Christian world, enriching the body of the Church with new kind of vocation to sanctity. In the eyes of the pagans of the fourth century, to say nothing of many modern attitudes toward contemplatives, the monk seemed to be a kind of madman suffering from misanthropy, oblivious of the fact that the human person is a social being made for civilization. The monk, however, insisted that he took all humanity with him to the desert where he felt himself bound up with the whole church and the whole world.

As monasticism progressed it took on different forms (e.g., the monks grouped into communities, or monasteries). Throughout Christian antiquity, Egypt never ceased to appear the chosen land of monasticism, though it began to spread throughout the Western world. When, by the end of the fourth century, it had come to Italy, Spain, Gaul, and Africa, this Latin monasticism was still fed directly from Eastern sources.

A rudimentary knowledge of monasticism's formative influence is important because private devotions and personal ascetical practices were, for the most part, inspired by monasticism. When a Christian living in the world wanted to lead a more intense religious life, quite naturally he looked to the monks to define the kind of life that he would try to imitate in due proportion. It was, moreover, the kind of life that the church prescribed for its public sinners during their period of expiation. It can be summed up in three words: prayer, fasting, alms.

Fasting was accompanied by a whole series of other austerities relating to sleep, clothes, comfort, and property. As a symbol of the whole, we may take the fact that some Christians gave up using the hot baths, the characteristic luxury of the Roman *dolce vita*.

The lesson to be drawn from early monasticism is that it is only in linking all asceticism with mysticism or union with God that we can avoid à faulty theological anthropology with its debasement of human nature and subsequent body-and-soul dichotomy. Where early monasticism did this, it flowered into impressive expressions of loving, God-directed lives. Where it failed to do this, we find well-intended but unhealthy excesses.

Handing-on Ascetical Practice in the Medieval Era

In trying to set forth the use, misuse, and disuse of fasting as a practice of the Christian religious life, one must deal with it in terms of its inner-connectedness with the different prayer-forms and the themes of mortification, detachment, and atonement/penance that fill the pages of Christian history. When one reads a volume on the Middle Ages, for example, one does not find a chapter on "fasting" which neatly and clearly traces the practice from A.D. 600-1500. It is necessary to glean bits from here and there as one reads about medieval thought, spiritual life, liturgical practice and private devotions. And that—even though it is more work—is good, because it prevents a practice like fasting from appearing "a way" unto itself, which it never is in Christian life. Hence, it is necessary in these next few pages to keep several related strands in hand all at the same time.

In the fifth and sixth centuries in Europe, when Italy, the seat of imperial power, was listing badly and threatening to go under from the impact of the barbarian invasions, the church had to come to grips with some important realities of survival. Christianity needs a certain level of culture, knowledge, and literature to survive. If the church was to prevent the West from becoming barbarian, it had to devise an effective structure for education.

Hence the appearance at the beginning of the sixth century of the episcopal school—the nucleus from which our universities were later to develop. Here the bishop provided his clergy with the knowledge needed to fulfill their duties. From this developed the priestly school. The Second Council of Vaison in 529 decreed that all priests in charge of a parish were to give a Christian education to young children.

The decree could be called the birth certificate of our primary Christian school. This educational innovation made general a kind of education in the Christian life that to this point had only been available in the cloisters. In these schools, episcopal or parish, a synthesis was forged between schoolmaster and spiritual director that safeguarded the integral handing-on of Christian doctrine and its application and expression in the religious practices of Christian living. In this way arose the general type of Christian education to which the church has remained attached to our present day.

It was a period of robust, rather simple faith. Devotion had assumed a less communal, more individual aspect, which means that for practices like fasting, the means-or-end tangle was an ever-present, ensnaring net. When preoccupation with personal salvation becomes obsessive, as it did during this time, it is not God and his goodness we are looking at, but ourselves and our own eternal well-being. "The feeling which seems to dominate," observe Jean Danielou and Henri Marou (in *The Christian Centuries*) of the fifth and sixth centuries, "is that of reverential fear inspired by the sovereign power of God and his Saints." The threat of punishment was a major argument used to move the people, which indicates that the focus was somewhat off-center, according to the evangelist St. John: "God is love and anyone who lives in love lives in God, and God lives in him. Love will come to its perfection in us when we can face the day of judgment without fear, because even in this world we have become as he is. In love there can be no fear, because even in this world we have become as he is. Fear is driven out by perfect love: because to fear is to expect punishment, and anyone who is afraid is still imperfect in love" (1 John 4:16-18).

Asceticism in the Middle Ages

Every generation of Christians has in essence the same spiritual life inasmuch as all have faith in the divine redeemer whose life and commandments they know from the scriptures and the teaching authority of the church. All live as Christians by virtue of the gifts of faith and grace, which are nourished by the sacraments. Yet, during the passage of the Christian centuries the forms of devotion and the rhythms of sacramental life have both developed and changed from century to century and country to country.

The sixth to the tenth centuries are known, in terms of the history of spirituality, as the "monastic" centuries. The monks, who in an ever-growing majority were following the Rule of St. Benedict, were the sole and almost ubiquitous representatives of a dedicated life. The monastic life was, in fact, regarded as the only recognized form of the fervent Christian life. It was still a flight from the prevailing evil of the world. There was no question of comparing the spiritual ideal of monasticism with that of clerics or fervent Christians; the monastic life *was* the fervent Christian life.

Gradually, however, the nature of the vocation changed. The monks became a class of "professional intercessors" for the rest of the people. The vehicle for their intercession was the liturgical service, a long and elaborate ceremonial of praise, which came to usurp personal sanctification as the raison d'être of the monk. Monastic asceticism became more and more the discipline of a life of liturgical prayer. The monastic ideal, particularly at Cluny (France), was less than that of the Rule, in which the monk advanced in love, humility, and obedience by means of all the duties of community life, and more that of the dedicated servant-intercessor who by means of an almost perpetual stream of vocal prayer and praise helped to form the earthly counterpart of the heavenly choir.

Traditional monastic doctrine reached its summit with the writings of St. Anselm, preceded by John of Fecamp and followed by Hugh of St. Victor. This developing spirituality is particularly pertinent for our discussion because it is, as we would say today, more holistic. That is, Anselm never proposes "stages" of spiritual life or gives a dichotomizing analysis of the natural and supernatural powers of the human person. Growth in holiness comes from a life of liturgical prayer, meditation and fraternal charity. Anselm does not speak in the categories of an "active" or "contemplative" vocation. One is left with the sense that union with God is available to all, and that all of human life is provided with divinity.

The single monastic tradition then split into a number of allied branches. In the eleventh century Romuald and Peter Damian led a return to the silent, solitary, and austere eremetical existence. The world was once again positively evil, and the ark of refuge, the second baptism, was monastic life. It must be made possible for everyone to share in it: clerics must become "regular," laypeople can, become monastic affiliates, knights and hospitallers can keep the monastic Rule, and all can use as a prayer shorter versions of the Holy Office.

In the twelfth century a rival spiritual teaching appeared from one of the schools, the Cistercians. They aimed primarily at recreating primitive conditions (those of the desert and the Rule), and while this implied austerity, it was also a call to freedom of spirit. The daily schedule became open, with more time for reading and prayer. This combination of an open horarium with simplicity and austerity brought with it a new flowering of mystical prayer. Bernard of Clairvaux throughout his works, which are full of directness of appeal and personal warmth, asserts once more the practical counsels and commands that develop the Christian and monastic virtues. In his context, fasting is clearly considered a means and a help to overcome all obstacles that prevent the Christian from loving God and neighbor. It is perfectly on-target as facilitating the growing experience of God in the Christian's life and of the person's growing unity with God. He directly invites to something higher, to a personal union of love with the Son, the Word of God, to the mystical experience in its plenitude.

Up to this time, the experiences of women mystics had played little part in the spiritual literature of the age, but in the twelfth century, when for the first time founders and abbots began to make provisions for the spiritual direction of nuns, women mystics and writers begin the long line that leads through so many saints to the mystics of our own day.

In 1215 the Fourth Lateran Council took cognizance for the first time of the laity and legislated for them. The tradition that the monastic ascesis was the only way to salvation was on the wane among the laity. David Knowles and Dimitri Obolensky note (in *The Christian Centuries*) that Wolfram von Eschenbach is sometimes indicated as the first writer to put forward the thoughts and ideals of a devout but foward-looking and original layman. No matter how one analyzes the causes and motives of the Crusades and those who took part in them, they are at least an evidence of the power of religious ideas over the minds of all the people of this age. The monastic and penitential ideal had sunk deeply into the consciousness of all classes. For the first time in Western Europe large urban groups were making their needs and tastes known, and devotions and practices were growing up (like the stations of the cross, the Christmas crib, and the rosary) which had no roots in the cloister.

While this age was yet very conscious of sin and judgment (the crucifix and the Last Judgment were the favorite motifs in churches great and small), Bernard of Clairvaux was both an instance and a cause of the growth of a more loving approach to the Savior and of a new emphasis on his human nature and human sympathies, especially in the mysteries of the incarnation and childhood. This was accompanied by a more tender devotion to his mother, seen as the maiden of the annuniciation, the young mother in the stable, the faith companion by the cross, the advocate at Cana and the mother of all the children of God redeemed by her son.

As a line of the *Desiderata* reads, "Beyond a wholesome discipline, be gentle with yourself." This statement implies that we need discipline in our lives to make us gentle and yet firm—to help us become the whole and holy people we were meant to be. But beyond this discipline, we need to be gentle with ourselves—understanding our limitations as human beings. God does not demand some Spartan perfection of us, only that we keep trying to love him. This spirit of asceticism allows us to see ourselves within the context of a loving God who speaks to us words of comfort and consolation. This is an asceticism of gentle temperance and discipline in which we become more like the loving God who calls us to share his love with a light and joyful heart.

The ideals of the age, with its love of poverty and preaching and the imitation of the human life of Christ, came together in the orders of friars: the Franciscans and the Dominicans. St. Francis of Assisi, with his identification with the suffering Redeemer, inspired a great army of followers to a new kind of self-dedication and self-sacrifice. "Franciscan piety" served to maintain an affective Christocentric devotion throughout the Middle Ages. The great Franciscan theologians reflect the message of Francis in two ways: they stand for the primacy of love, looking to the love of God rather than to the truth and knowledge of God as the key to the universe; and they regard theology as primarily the guide to a life that leads to the ecstatic vision of God. All learning is in fact directed toward the love of God.

While it would be an undue simplification to say that the Franciscans aimed at changing the heart while the Dominicans were concerned with enlightening the mind, Thomas Aquinas's presentation of the theological virtues, of the infused moral virtues, of the gifts of the Holy Spirit, and of the contemplative life lie behind the classical ascetical and mystical doctrines of the Dominican order and molded the expressions of its saints. Tauler, a celebrated Dominican teaching in the fourteenth century, urged all his audiences to aim at a life of mystical experience. And to be sure, there were during this era a remarkable number of sane and impressive mystical groups, such as the mystics of the Rhineland and a series of spiritual writers in England who have borne the conventional name of "the English Mystics."

The traditional stream of spiritual teaching was to become familiar to multitudes of readers throughout the centuries in the writings of Dante. The traditional doctrine of the contemplative life found prophets and preachers among the laity. In England it was the poet William Langland; in Italy, Catherine of Siena; and in Sweden, Birgitta.

It is significant that these themes were picked up by and further disseminated to the laity who were immersed in "the real world," because Christian asceticism is only of value if accompanied by a positive acceptance and regard for the created order, a sense of responsibility for the world and fidelity to temporal tasks.

Only when Christian asceticism is lived free of a one-sided anthropology that views with suspicion the body, sex, marriage, and worldly matters in general, will it become clear that ascetism and mysticism are simply two aspects of the Christian life that cannot be separated. An attentive eye has been kept upon the mystics in our survey because if asceticism and mysticism merge into one another and are basically inseparable, asceticism cannot be regarded as a subject to be studied on its own, as has been done from the seventeenth century onward.

"Fooling With Works" and the Reformation

The Reformation was a many-sided event, not merely a religious one. Humanism, philosophy, politics, and economics contributed largely to its origin, form, and content. It was part of the shift in European thought and experience that had begun in the fourteenth century.

Nonetheless, at its core it was a religious movement and a theological event in the great trends launched by Luther, in whom it reached its fullest expression. Thus the Reformation is an important chapter in the history of theology and religious experience. Its impact on world history was the result of the condition of the Church itself.

In theology, Thomism was still active here and there, but was on the whole in decline. It was the heyday of nominalism, which represented a fundamental critique of the existing philosophical and theological tradition by maintaining that the metaphysical notion of the "universal" was a *flatus vocis*—an "empty word" that has no relation to reality. Nominalism influenced persistently the thought of the Middle Ages and even of modern times. It subjected the faith to logic-chopping in a decidedly nonbiblical form of thought.

As regards fasting, a vast system of casuistry had developed, touching upon questions of permitted and forbidden food, indulgences and dispensions. There was a perilous Pelagianizing* of justification, which Luther was to denounce as a "fooling with works." His criticism of the exaggerated emphasis placed upon the role of human forces in salvation was warranted.

When fasting or other exercises of self-denial are undertaken to make reparation and penance, they have the character of a sacrifice. The deepest sense of fasting in this context lies in the recognition that God is the absolute and holy and supreme Lord of all creation, and by sacrifice one makes a concrete act of dedication to him and to his service. But this must be done by virtue of the one and only valid sacrifice: that of Christ. It must not be subconsciously taken as one's own meritorious religious achievement. As such, it is without value and to be rejected, religiously speaking. Any asceticism that wishes to call itself Christian must be grounded in the consciousness of our indebtedness; it becomes Christian in the strict sense only within the explicit context of sin, the divine judgment on sin, and redemption through the cross of Christ. If fasting had no relationship to this context, it would be constantly in danger of striving after personal achievement in spite of the knowledge that the help of God's grace is indispensable.

What had happened to the Mass by this time is a perfect example of piety gone wrong. The sacraments had come to be envisaged in a very material way, e.g., Mass was a "good work" of finite value, whose fruits were distributed piecemeal to the hearers. The result was the effort to have as many Masses said and heard as possible. Church life, in general, was often almost exclusive preoccupation with gaining foreseeable merits through the accomplishments of varius precepts. The doctrine of indulgences was seen in a very dubious light, with the Pope "dispensing" from the "treasury" of the church.

The credibility of the church had suffered. Theology lost its substance inasmuch as it departed from the central questions like redemption, faith, and justification. The discussion of the church as a sacramental and spiritual institution was almost entirely lacking. Clerical life fell short of true Christian standards on all levels and

---

*Pelagianism was a belief that denied original sin and over-emphasized man's ability, apart from grace, to attain salvation.

became characterized by worldliness, pleasure-seeking, immorality, lack of pastoral zeal, and simony. The style of life of the Renaissance itself was an important factor, for it was markedly hedonistic and had a wide influence on Christendom.

A reformation in the sense of a radical critique had become historically unavoidable. The just and central demands of the reformers had a rightful place *within* the church. "Reformation" was a watchword of a religious movement for renewal that did not aim at creating a breach; Luther used the word to sum up his program of *metanoia*, the restoration of the ancient Christian truth by serious attention to the living word of the Bible. The protagonists saw the Reformation as the recovery of the pure revelation of primitive Christianity, while the Catholic Church of the time saw it mainly as a rejection of Christian truth. The Council of Trent, 1545-1563, was called to reform the church in the face of the spread of Protestantism. Its doctrinal utterances were made from a defensive stance, with a view to what it believed were Protestant errors. Its position, therefore, made almost impossible a *rapprochement* between the two bodies.

But now it may be said that wherever the fault lay, it was a *felix culpa* since in many ways the reformers succeeded in presenting the pure Gospel to Christians and reasserting the ancient Catholic truth. The goal of the Reformation, a purified Christianity in the one church, was not attained. This goal is a permanent task. Though it cannot be brought about solely by our efforts, it will not happen without them. Faith and courage are needed, and the selflessness of love and service.

The Individualist Emphasis in Piety and Morality

In the perspective of the great movements of the human spirit, Jansenism may be seen as a reaction, in line with that of the Reformation. A movement with the seventeenth and eighteenth centuries, it represents one effort to solve the problem with which all Christian life is faced: that of reconciling the fundamental antagonisms inherent in Christianity. On the one hand, for example, one is to love and care for the world that has been entrusted to us, and on the other, there are aspects of the world which one is to resist. There is the necessity, on the one hand, of working out one's salvation responsibly while, on the other hand, realizing that it is a freely bestowed gift. In the eventual judgment of Christendom, this great problem, which is at the basis of all the others—how to reconcile divine grace which is absolutely gratuitous and beyond merit with personal human responsibility—could not be solved along Jansenistic lines. Its crippled anthropology saw the body as basically evil and the pleasures of the world as intrinsically incompatible with sanctity.

In his spirituality of the movement for reform, Luther sought to underline the irreplaceable individuality of the believer. Until the time of the Reformation, spirituality was combined with the outward and the interior life of the church. But as the church sealed itself off in defensive reaction, people looked inwards. This individualist emphasis in piety and morality expressed itself in both positive and negative ways in the nineteenth century.

The century preceding our own is much-maligned for being an age of religious decadence and of mounting success for irreligion and immorality, but when one looks below the surface one discerns a spiritual revival for which it would be hard to find a parallel down the centuries. On the positive side, there was a remarkable revival of religious orders and congregations, many outward signs of individual and collective piety, the beginnings of a new outpouring of devotional literature, the expansion of charitable and other associations of every description. Underlying all of this, one can only assume that a more than ordinary devotion and generosity among the mass of the faithful was operating.

A profound and lasting change took place during the middle years of the nineteenth century. The austere and undemonstrative piety characteristic of the preceding generations, confined in practice to an elite, gave way to a piety more accessible to the masses. Devotion came to focus increasingly on the suffering Christ, opening his heart so full of love toward us (the devotion to the Sacred Heart).

On the unfortunate side of this new devotional trend religious practice focused, often with a want of discretion that helped to deepen the gulf between Catholics and Protestants, on the Virgin and on certain saints beloved by the people. These devotions were often insipid and infantile, as can be judged from the many artless hymns and a body of devotional literature whose good intentions were no protection against mediocrity and bad taste. As was the case with the practice of fasting, the accent was too often on the observance of a code, a code more moral than religious and one enjoining an individualist and legalistic type of morality. The stress on individual moral actions narrowed still further the perspective of the many faithful who had already lost contact with the Bible and the liturgy. The lack of an overall perspective as to where these individual practices should fit in, the absence of doctrinal clarity, resulted in a general tendency to load up with minute rules and regulations. The spirituality of the period, largely perduring up to the mid-twentieth century, for want of this firm foundation, often degenerated into prescription. Witness this excerpt on Fasting, published in 1967, in the *New Catholic Encyclopedia*:

> . . . Nondigestible matter, such as paper, fingernails, or tobacco, does not break the fast. Any digestible thing in a solid state when taken orally is considered food, even if it liquefies in the mouth before being swallowed, e.g., a caramel. Ordinary chewing gum probably does not break the fast; nor is it broken by what comes from within the mouth, e.g., blood from the gums or food remaining in the teeth from a previous meal. The fast is not broken by what is taken into the stomach along with saliva, nor by what is taken along with breathing, e.g., insects blown into the mouth . . . .

Not that externals are not important in their own right, but a one-sided emphasis on just *doing* things without a corresponding emphasis on *reasons* and *values* will produce a mechanical, external compliance. Is this to say that past Catholic practice in this regard was meaningless? No, but it is to say that spiritual exercises and private devotions don't exist for themselves. They exist to help us express and grow in our faith, our hope, our love, our gratitude. They exist to help us become more genuinely open to the acceptance of God's will, to assist us in looking upon the events of our lives with faith, and to enable us to make ourselves more and more aware of God as the deepest reality of our lives. The value of any particular practice is related to its ability or effectiveness in doing that. When we have lost the spirit of the practice and are engaged in only a mindless repetition of its form, it is perhaps better than it is lost for a time so that it can be rediscovered again and embraced once more— with feeling and understanding.

Fasting in the Christian Churches Today

Today we Christians are in the peculiar position of being inspired by the fasting disciplines of others. The absence of a practice of fasting among Christians is a source of scandal to the Muslim world. The fasting experience of a whole nation is a deep witness to the solidarity of the people in their faith and tradition, as exemplified by the corporate, month-long fast of Ramadan in Algeria. When one hears, however, that while the Muslims keep carefully the fast that the law requires until sundown, and then proceed to stuff themselves after the sun has gone down, one wonders whether they have fallen into the same well of legalism from which Catholics are now trying to crawl out.

In an era where churches and nations and religious orders and ethnic groups are returning to their sources, we are impressed to see the primitive natives of Venezuela holding tight to their age-old custom of fasting as an expression that their spirit is stronger than any appetite. And we are impressed by the Mormon practice of fasting from the lunch meal of Saturday to the lunch meal of Sunday, (one misses supper and breakfast) on the first weekend of every month, in order to devote themselves more effectively to prayer, reflection, and charity.

In the Anglican and main-line Protestant churches today, the question of fasting is left to the individual member. Each is to decide for him or herself whether one will fast, and how. In the Anglican Communion, the more important fast days are recommended in the Book of Common Prayer. The list includes all Fridays, Lent, the Ember Days (Ember days originated at Rome about the fifth century, probably as Christian replacements for seasonal festivals of agrarian cults. They were observances of penance, thanksgiving and petition for divine blessing on the various seasons. These days were observed four times a year: on the Wednesday, Friday, and Saturday following the third Sunday of September) and certain vigils, but merely enjoins a special measure of devotion and abstinence on these days, laying down no precise law for their observance, the details of which are left to the discretion of local ecclesiastical authorities. Some Lutherans urge that a fast be kept before partaking of the Lord's Supper, but leave the method of keeping it to the devotion of the one fasting.

What this Lutheran approach highlights is a *cultic* asceticism that has not only been found in Christianity but in all formal religions. Cultic asceticism touches on abstinence and acts preparatory to one's participation in the mysteries of divine cult and liturgy. In the Old Testament, this consists in fasting, vigils, sexual abstinence, washings, the offering of animals, and that of incense.

It is in the Eastern Church that we find the cultic asceticism of fasting more in evidence than anywhere. Days observed by fasting and abstinence have been so numerous at different times that the total has been as high as 180 days in the course of a year! And all of them come as preparatory acts for one's participation in the liturgical mysteries. In addition to the great, or major Lent, three other "Lents" have been observed in the Greek Church: the Lent of the Holy Apostles (June 16-28), Mary's Lent (August 1-14), and the Lent preceding Christmas (November 15-December 24). It was also observed on, besides these four extended seasons of fasting, the vigils of the Epiphany, St. John Baptist's Day, Holy Cross Day, and every Wednesday and Friday. Today, much of such cultic preparation has been relegated to one's individual inspiration, and the Church members as a whole do not generally enter into any common cultic preparation in such an ascetical manner.

Orthodox Christians fast because Jesus fasted and taught his disciples to fast. Their clearly stated purpose is to gain mastery over oneself and to liberate oneself from passions. According to the universal witness of the saints, fasting is an excellent means of gaining the fruit of the Holy Spirit in one's life; also, Jesus taught that certain sins cannot be overcome except "by prayer and fasting."

Orthodox Christians do *not* fast because they think it "pleases God" not to eat; the lenten hymns of the church remind them that "the Devil also never eats." The do *not* fast in order to "punish" or "afflict" themselves. They do *not* fast as a means of "repairing" sinful deeds (since the only reparation for sin is Christ's love, revealed in his crucifixion).

Fasting in preparation for Easter is an ancient and holy custom of the Orthodox. This activity includes, besides dietary fasting, abstinence from the normal activities of one's life: entertainment such as television and movies, sexual relations between wives and husbands, etc. This "makes time" for activities for which we often "have no time": church services, study of the New Testament and reading of good books, visiting the sick and shut-ins, etc. According to the teaching of Jesus, all this is to be done *in secret*. The rule is a strict one, and each must fulfill it according to his own desire and ability.

The following rules of fasting for Orthodox Christians are taken from *The Lenten Triodion*:

(1) During the week between the Sunday of the Publican and the Pharisee and that of the Prodigal Son, there is a general dispensation from all fasting. Meat and animal products may be eaten all the time.

(2) In the following week, often termed *Carnival Week*, the usual fast is kept on Wednesday and Friday. Otherwise, there is no special fasting.

(3) In the week before Lent, meat is forbidden, but eggs, cheese and other dairy products may be eaten on all days, including Wednesday and Friday.

(4) On weekdays (Monday to Friday inclusive) during the seven weeks of Lent, there are restrictions both on the *number* of meals taken daily and on the *types of food* permitted. But when a meal is allowed, there is no fixed limitation on the *quantity* of food to be eaten.

a) On weekdays of the *first* week, fasting is particularly severe. According to the strict observance, in the course of the five initial days of Lent, only two meals are eaten, one on Wednesday and the other on Friday, in both cases after the Liturgy of the Presanctified Gifts. On the other three days, those who have the strength are encouraged to keep an absolute fast; those for whom this proves impracticable may eat on Tuesday and Thursday (but not, if possible, on Monday), in the evening after Vespers, when they may take bread and water, or perhaps tea or fruit juice (but not a cooked meal). *It should be added at once that in practice today these rules are commonly relaxed.* At the meals on Wednesday and Friday *xerophagy* is prescribed; literally, this means "dry eating." Strictly interpreted, it signifies that we may eat only vegetables cooked with water and salt, and also such things as fruit, nuts, bread and honey. In practice, sea food is also allowed on days of xerophagy; likewise vegetable margarine and corn or other vegetable oil, not made from olives. But the following are excluded: meat, animal products (cheese, milk, butter, eggs, lard, drippings), fish (i.e., fish with backbone), oil (i.e., olive oil) and wine (i.e., all alcoholic drinks).

b) On weekdays (Monday to Friday inclusive) on the *second, third, fourth, fifth* and *sixth weeks*, one meal a day is permitted, to be taken in the afternoon following Vespers, and at this one meal xerophagy is to be observed.

c) *Holy Week.* On the *first three days*, one meal a day is taken with xerophagy; but some try to keep a complete fast on these days, or else they eat only uncooked foods, as on the opening days of the first week.

On *Holy Thursday* one meal is eaten, with wine and oil (i.e., olive oil).

On *Great Friday* those who have the strength follow the practice of the Early Church and keep a total fast. Those unable to do this may eat bread, with a little water, tea or fruit juice, but not until sunset, or at any rate until after the veneration of the Epitaphion at Vespers.

On *Holy Saturday* there is in principle no meal, since according to the ancient practice after the end of the Liturgy of St. Basil the faithful remained in church for the reading of *The Acts of the Apostles*, and for their sustenance were given a little bread and dried fruit, with a cup of wine. If, as usually happens now, they return home for a meal, they may use wine but not oil; for on this one Saturday, alone among the Saturdays of the year olive oil is not permitted.

The rule of xerophagy is relaxed on the following days: on *Saturdays and Sundays* in Lent, with the exception of Holy Saturday, two main meals may be taken in the usual way, around mid-day and in the evening, with wine and olive oil; but meat, animal products and fish are now allowed. On the *Feast of the Annunciation (25 March)* and *Palm Sunday*, fish is permitted as well as wine and oil, but meat and animal products are not allowed. If the Feast of Annunciation falls on the first four days of Holy Week, wine and oil are permitted but not fish. If it falls on Great Friday or Holy Saturday, wine is permitted, but not fish or oil.

It has always been held that these rules of fasting should be relaxed in the case of anyone elderly or in poor health. In present-day practice, even for those in good health, the full strictness of the fast is usually mitigated. Only a few Orthodox today attempt to keep a total fast on Monday, Tuesday and Thursday in the first week, or on the first three days in Holy Week. On weekdays—except, perhaps, during the first week of Holy Week—it is now common to eat two cooked meals daily instead of one. From the second until the sixth weeks, many Orthodox use wine, and perhaps oil also, on Tuesdays and Thursdays, and less commonly on Mondays as well. Permission is often given to eat fish in these weeks.

Personal factors need to be taken into account, as for example the situation of an isolated Orthodox living in the same household as non-Orthodox, or obliged to take meals in a factory or school cafeteria. In cases of uncertainty each is to seek the advice of his or her spiritual father.

The literature on fasting among Orthodox Christians emphasizes that at all times it is essential to bear in mind "that you are not under the law but under grace" (Romans 6:14) and that "the letter kills, but the spirit gives life" (2 Corinthians 3:6). The rules of fasting, while they need to be taken seriously, are not to be interpreted with dour and pedantic legalism: "for the kingdom of God is not food and drink, but righteousness and peace and joy in the Holy Spirit" (Romans 14:17).

Some special attention must be given to that group of Christians who, more than any other, has been associated (up until recently) with the practice of fasting in the popular contemporary mind: Roman Catholics. It has been 400 years since the Christians in this tradition experienced anything quite like the past two decades. Roman Catholics have felt disconcerted as they watched the disappearance of so many familiar landmarks—one of which was a practice by which they were identified: the Friday abstinence.

Why did so many Catholic devotional practices and spiritual-life exercises decline after the Second Vatican Council (1962-1965)? One answer will not suffice. There are several: A misguided eagerness in implementing the changes called for by Vatican II. Changes in living habits in an on-the-go modern society with more to do, see, and choose from. Changes in values, behavioral styles, ways of doing and seeing and comprehending things. And, perhaps most of all, the exaggerated importance given to traditional devotional practices in the pre-Council, Latin-liturgy era. But even that needs to be put into perspective. When you consider that these practices of piety were the only things that the laity could actually participate in or experience without the need for an explanation or a translation, it's pretty difficult to condemn people for taking them seriously.

It is hard to trace cause and effect very precisely in a matter such as this because where people are involved in changes of vast proportion and consequence, many different causes come together to create many effects. Perhaps the core of the controversy today is best reached simply by saying that there had to be a change in *emphasis*. A greater emphasis on Scripture. More of a central focus upon Christ in the liturgy. More of a positive view of salvation as already here, not something that has to be earned. More of an appreciation for the Holy Spirit in our lives. More of an underlining of the importance and dignity of the role of the laity. More of a joyful vision of the Christian vocation to "bear fruit in charity for the good of the world."

As was noted earlier, the Western Catholic spirituality of the modern era, for want of the firm foundation of doctrinal clarity, often degenerated into prescription. Nowhere is this more evident than the recent Roman Catholic practice of fasting.

Until 1917 the general law required the faithful to fast on all the days of Lent except Sunday; on Wednesdays, Fridays, and Saturdays of the Ember weeks, and on the vigils of Christmas, Pentecost, Assumption, and All Saints. By custom in many places, the Wednesdays and Fridays of Advent were also fast days. By fasting was understood the taking of only one meal a day with abstinence from meat, eggs and milk products. Abstinence without fast was observed on all Fridays and Saturdays throughout the year.

Local dispensations often softened these general prohibitions. In the U.S., for example, the bishops obtained a number of dispensations that changed the face of things considerably. In 1837, the fathers of the Third Provincial Council of Baltimore obtained a dispensation from the custom of fasting on the Wednesdays and Fridays of Advent. An indult dispensing from the Saturday abstinence had already been granted and was renewed in 1840. In 1886, Leo XIII granted a Lenten indult to the U.S. that permitted the taking of meat, eggs, and milk products at the principal meal on all days except Wednesdays and Fridays and Holy Saturday. In 1941, Pius XII granted to all the bishops of the world the power to dispense entirely from fast and abstinence except on Ash Wednesday and Good Friday. The Pope must have thought he had gone too far, because in 1949, some restrictions on this faculty were imposed, namely that abstinence must be observed on all Fridays of the year; fast and abstinence on Ash Wednesday, Good Friday, and the vigils of Assumption and Christmas. In constant use until 1951 was the "workingman's law" that permitted flesh meat to be eaten in those circumstances of place and person in which the common law of abstinence could not be observed without real difficulty. This concession benefitted not only the individual workingman but applied also to his family.

In 1951 a bishops' committee drew up a formula of uniform norms that became the basis for diocesan regulations in the U.S.:

Fasting and Abstaining

1. Fasting

   a) On days of fast only one full meal is allowed. Two other meals without meat may be taken according to one's need. But together these two meals should not equal a full meal.

   b) Those bound to fast: all those between 21 (completed) and 59 (completed) are bound to fast unless exempted or dispensed. In case of doubt about exemption or dispensation a parish priest or confessor should be asked.

2. Abstinence

   a) Partial abstinence: on days of partial abstinence meat and products made from meat may be taken only once a day. Days of partial abstinence are always days of fast and those who are not obliged to fast are not thereby excused from abstinence.

   b) Complete abstinence: on days of complete abstinence no meat or products made from meat may be taken.

   c) Those bound to abstain: all those seven years of age and older unless exempted or dispensed.

71

3. Days of Fast and Abstinence

   a) Fast only: all weekdays of Lent except Ash Wednesday, Fridays, Ember Wednesday and Saturday and Holy Saturday.

   b) Fast and partial abstinence: Ember Wednesday and Saturday, Vigil of Pentecost and Eve of All Saints (unless this latter is a Friday).

   c) Fast and complete abstinence: Fridays of Lent, Ember Fridays, Ash Wednesday, Holy Saturday, Eve of the Assumption (August 14), Eve of Christmas, and Eve of All Saints (October 31), if it falls on a Friday.

   d) Abstinence only: all Fridays of the year except Fridays of Lent and Ember Friday.

Finally, in the apostolic constitution *Poenitemini* of Pope Paul VI (Feb. 17, 1966), there was a total reorganization of ecclesiastical discipline with regard to fasting and abstinence. Abstinence from meat and meat products, it said, was to be observed on every Friday, and fast as well as abstinence on Ash Wednesday and Good Friday. The constitution changed the age at which one should begin to observe abstinence from seven to fourteen years, and changed the age at which one ceases to be obliged by the law of fasting to the completion of one's sixtieth year. Most significantly, Pope Paul authorized bishops' conferences to adapt the laws of fasting and abstinence to suit modern conditions and to emphasize prayer and works of charity as substitutes for previous practices of abstinence and fasting.

In November of that same year, the U.S. bishops did adapt the laws. They weren't saying that fasting isn't important any more. The message behind the seeming sell-out to the modern spirit of convenience and indulgence was that fasting was *so* important that it had to be rescued from the legalism, minimalism, and externalism into which it had fallen. The bishops followed up the Pope's document with a pastoral statement which recommended that Catholics continue *voluntarily* to observe *some* (note: not necessarily fasting) acts of penance on *all* Fridays of the year. While Friday

72

abstinence from meat was itself not going to be required by law (except during Lent), Fridays were singled out as days on which we should try to give special expression to our everyday call to love by entering into some other-related activities: "It would bring great glory to God and good to souls," they wrote, "if Fridays found our people doing volunteer work in hospitals, visiting the sick, serving the needs of the aged and lonely, instructing the young in the faith, participating as Christians in community affairs, and meeting obligations to families, friends, neighbors, and parish with special zeal. . . ."

My perception is, however, that most Catholics have a sense that something was taken away and that nothing positive was put in its place. Hindsight evaluation indicates that when the changes were being interpreted to the people on the parish level, this positive emphasis should have received a lot more energy and attention. Chances are that most of the membership doesn't know their religious leaders ever said that abstinence and fast should be *substituted* wholly or in part with other forms of penitence, works of charity, and exercises of piety.

Neither Pope Paul nor the U.S. bishops intended to deemphasize the need for fasting. Rather, they underlined it in red. But they did it in a way that Roman Catholics haven't been reared to appreciate, i.e., by *removing* the laws instead of putting more laws there. They challenged people to junk their unreal compart-mentalizations and to rediscover the spirit of it. Recognizing that the practices of fast and abstinence had become like sleepwalking for most Catholics, they yelled: "Wake up, and look where you're going!" Since sleepwalking is never the most effective means of getting where you want to go, the bishops called upon their people to see that the Lenten fast and the Friday abstinence were not necessarily the most effective means of practicing penance. Visiting old Mrs. Meier in the nursing home might be a lot harder and actually do some good.

Lent itself was in danger of being strangled by the tentacles of legalism. The Mardi Gras pig-out and the Easter Sunday fat-attack symbolize, on one level, an unreal confining of a means of spiritual growth to the six weeks of Lent. But fasting isn't just for Lent—it's for Christian *life*! When it is bottled up and stamped "must be disposed of" by such and such a date (like the milk in the refrigerator), it has not been understood *why* fasting is recommended at all.

73

Something important happened, a significant shift occurred. Whereas the Roman Catholic Church used to stress *both* the need for and the how-to details of this spiritual-life tool, it was now choosing just to reaffirm the need for and leave the details up to its members. It asked them to be adults in the faith; to act responsibly, i.e., with awareness; to use the tools of the spiritual life that fit their needs and situation and that express their inner conversion of heart.

The era of imposed fasting is only a memory now for *all* Christians. Fasting today is an exercise of freedom and of spiritual exploration. We have come full circle. We have the luxury of approaching fasting as the early Christians did, with an attitude of individual liberty. T. S. Eliot once wrote: "The end of all our journeying is to end up where we began and to recognize the place for the first time."

What was true of the early Christians, however, and is not yet true of us, is that frequent fasting in liberty was considered *normal* as an ascetical means to express sorrow for sin, to control concupiscence, and to intercede powerfully before God.

4

Much of What It Would Be Useful for You To Know About Fasting But Which You Were Never Before Interested Enough to Ask

*Until someone has experienced the question,
it's not likely that the answer will be interiorized.*

—Teacher's Manual

As we've seen, the art of the why, the how, and the when of fasting has been largely lost in the Judaeo-Christian tradition. The habit and practice have withered along with the sense of God. The wisdom slipped away from us like the quiet dying-in-the-night of a grandfather. The language became ossified and regarded like Old English or Latin. The vision that breathed life into the tradition of fasting developed a cataract.

One of the culprits seems to have been overlegislation of the value. So you can be very sure that I'm not going to turn around and try to lay out a whole set of new rules. We celebrated the passing of that era in the last chapter. All that is offered here is extended in the spirit of suggestion and counsel for those who are seeking and interested.

What is presented here is also liberally laced with what we know about fasting from the scientific study of it. Fasting should certainly not be conducted *un*-scientifically, that is, in a way that ignores or goes against what we have learned through medical science. With this information it is possible to provide a secure framework within which the faster may seek the Lord with every assurance that what one is doing is advancing his or her own health as well as the state of the relationship with God. If something is not good for *you*, it is an illusion to think it is good for your relationship with God. We were made to be healthy and happy.

This chapter breaks the task of getting down to the nitty-gritty into four parts: The mindset that should characterize the fast if the fst is intended to be an act of faith, hope, and love; some preliminary questions that ought to calm anxieties; the how of fasting (which includes the how long and the how to end it); and the when, in which section my own thinking takes the form of some concrete proposals.

The Mindset

One of the fundamental objectives of this book is to assist in the renewal of our appreciation for fasting as a religious act. As each of us developed our moral sense through the interactions of home, friends and school, we learned that the "why" of what we did made a big difference in terms of how that act was responded to. Why did you wake your little brother—because you thought the house was on fire or because you were mad at him? Why does he get to do that and you don't—is there some special reason or is he just the teacher's favorite? Why do you want to get married—because she's pregnant or because you love her? Why did you fire your gun—was it in self-defense or because you came home upset that night? The *why* that lies behind our behavior is directly linked to what's in our head and heart, and since the two of those working in harmony is what gives meaning to our actions, the reason *why* we do something deserves careful attention.

As we have seen, there are all kinds of reasons—valid ones in their own right—why people abstain from food. What are some of the reasons why I might want to abstain from food as part of my relationship with God?

Principally, because fasting can be a focus of the heart if entered into with a particular mind-and-heart set. Always when we voluntarily go without food, it is because something else is more important to us. It might be an early departure, a slim waistline, or a feeling of physical well-being. But it might also be because I want to say in a very real way: God, you are number one for me; you are more important to me than life itself, which food symbolizes for me. With this fast, I want to send you that message. I also want to impress upon myself that you are at the center of life's meaning, and it is therefore important for me regularly to renew that realization in very real and concrete ways, which succeed in bringing the truth home to me. The focus away from food (and what it symbolizes as one of the goods of existence that we need) to God is deliberate. Yes these other goods are important. Yes I need them. But all the needs in my life, if traced down to their deepest core, are rooted in my single, greatest need: for fulfillment from the hand of my Creator. From time to time I can forget just which needs are the most important, and my priorities can become all mixed up. Fasting cuts through the drift and ambiguity like a meat cleaver coming down on a butcher's table. It is a concrete, decisive act that says: "You, Lord, are the still point in my turning world, and please don't let me ever forget it. For you, I will upset my routine today of three meals because you are the God I worship, not my routine (which becomes all too important for me sometimes). For you I will give up meeting my friends for lunch today because, even though I need them and like them very much, the love and acceptance I need from them is only a reflection of the love and acceptance I need from you. For you I will live with these hunger pangs today and let them speak to me of my deepest hungers: our hearts are restless, Lord, until they rest in you."

Men and women from Jesus to Augustine to Aquinas to Teresa of Avila to Martin Luther to John Calvin to John Henry Newman to Martin Luther King all discovered that abstaining from food freed them to focus upon God with fresh intensity and opened avenues of spiritual perception and understanding that were not available during the rush of routine living. They found that as they focused upon God by the deliberate discipline of fasting, that God focused upon them and spoke to their hearts with clarity of direction and quickening of spirit.

God is all about us, like air, waiting upon our freedom for the invitation to come within, waiting upon the least sign of openness on our part to deepen the communion with himself, but our daily flurry of activity and interaction keeps his presence from our awareness. During times of fasting, however, the simple fact that we're not walking out of the shop or office toward the restaurant, the simple sensations emitted by an empty stomach, will serve to remind us of God's presence in our lives, because it was not for this that we deliberately determined to disrupt our routine today. Meals *are* important in so many ways—as social event, as a needed break from work, as nutrition—and when we voluntarily forego this as part of the language of our relationship with God it takes on the meaning that we are willing to set aside all else that would interfere with seeking God wholeheartedly. Eating symbolizes that which is most essential to us: life and growth. By setting this aside to seek God, we are declaring that he is more important and essential a source of life and growth than anything else. "I have esteemed the words of his mouth more than my necessary food" (Job 23:12).

When our focus of heart is right, we are like a radar screen that is tracking well. And when our focus is not clear, this, too, has a way of showing in the countenance, attitudes, and even the conditions of our bodies. Our hearts were made to enjoy God and they flourish in his presence. Nothing else can satisfy them. When the heart is not aimed at him who alone can fulfill it, it is like a disoriented homing pigeon, or a teen-ager traveling in a foreign land, showing signs of homesickness.

The spirit of fasting as an act of faith is captured in Psalm 16:

I have set the Lord ever before me:
Because He is at my right hand,
I shall not be moved.
Therefore my heart is glad
And my soul rejoices;
my flesh, too, abides in confidence.
You will show me the path of life:
In your presence is fullness of joy,
At your right hand are pleasures forevermore.

Since God is our well-being, when we are rightly focused on him, all else falls into perspective. The balanced life that flows naturally from this perspective is a path of joy—not the kind of cart-wheeling, yelling, screaming "school's-out-for-the-year!" joy, but the deep, peaceful serenity that comes from being rooted in a solid place. It is only when fasting is seen as a focus upon God as our rock, our fortress, our shelter in time of stress, that we can understand why fasting is characterized by a quiet joy:

Thus says the Lord of hosts: the fast of the fourth month, and the fast of the fifth, and the fast of the seventh, and the fast of the tenth, shall be to the house of Judah joy and gladness, cheerful feasts; therefore, love and truth and peace (Zechariah 8:19).

Fasting is definitely an act of worship. When we go to church each week, one of the things that happens is the restoration of a sense of perspective. The petty grievances, self-preoccupations, and the cares of this life that have marked our week are put into perspective as we consciously enter into confessing at worship that God is bigger and more important than all else that concerns us. We glorify him with our praises, our songs, our listening, our silent prayer—in short, by giving him our attention.

This is the same dynamic that is going on in fasting. It serves to make us stop dissipating our attention and return to focus on God. It calls a halt to our scattered activities and restores perspective. It makes us realize all over again that basic to all our activity is relationship with God. We know how easy it is to get off-center and be carried away on detours. Fasting pulls us up short. It's a map check that puts us back on the right road. In the Sermon on the Mount, Jesus gave us a look through a viewfinder that operated according to God's perspective. In it, we see that God is at the center of the picture, and all we do is meant to spring from our heart-relationship with him.

The Aim of Christian Fasting

Growth in our relationship with God is not measured, therefore, by the difficulty of the practices performed, but rather by now unswervingly we direct everything toward God.

A basic reason why so many of us good people are not enjoying a deeper intimacy in our relationship with the Lord is that there is a kind of double-fault in our approach. Most of our efforts are in the negative (not doing wrong things), and are performed with a legalistic mindset (practicing a certain number of right things). What needs to happen is a radical transformation at the well-springs of our daily activity that keeps us in touch with the indwelling Trinity who seeks to guide us toward our ultimate end. From an ever-deepening sense of God's presence with us comes the flexibility to move in every event toward the direction of God.

The good of every ascetical practice in the Christian life is to move us irrevocably away from self-centeredness to a God-centering. It is a singleness of vision that makes God and his will for us more and more the only criterion of our choices. ". . . if your eye is sound, your whole body will be filled with light" (Matthew 6:22).

The point at which our human freedom reaches its peak is when we, having experienced in our daily lives the abundant love of God for us, move freely, spontaneously, and with a spirit of improvisation to return God's love. Thus a person may freely offer to God a day's fasting out of a sheer desire to love God. Such a motive represents the quintessential religious act: a desire to return love by love. It is not any hardship or sacrifice involved that is ennobling, but the motive to offer God a free-gift return out of love.

The authentic aim of fasting as our act of Christian asceticism is always to lead us to a deeper union in love with God and appreciation for his universe and all its creatures which is, as we have noted earlier, the essence of mysticism.

"Asceticism and mysticism," writes George Maloney, one of the few acknowledged masters of the spiritual life in North America, "cannot be separated just as the seed and the fruit contain each other in a total entity. Yet fruit cannot be attained without the asceticism of the seed dying and the new life cultivated slowly through hard work, sun, rain, and wind. This dying process, of course, is not what produces fruit. Only the spirit can bring forth the fruit of the Father which is His life shared with us."

We need not, then, be afraid or feel presumptious to speak of union with God. It is what we are meant for.

Fasting in Secret

One of the ways God will know that our fast is intended for him is that he's the only one who knows! As we focus upon God through prayer and fasting, he looks upon our hearts with increased attention, examining the "why" of what we're doing. As anyone would who has taken the initiative in having a relationship with someone, he wants to know if our driving by his house is because we want to see him or whether we're just going by there on the way to somewhere else. He wants to know whether our fasting represents a knocking on *his* door. Rather than counting the meals that we've missed, he's probably looking right into our hearts. Many of the people of his Son's day had lost the art of being real with him. Their religion was marked by a lot of public show, but a peep behind the curtain showed it was clearly vaudeville. They dressed and acted in ways that would hopefully portray them to be deeply religious. But God is a penetrating critic and the show has yet to be put together that can convince him it's got a lot of substance if it's really founded on tinsel and glitter. When he sees an act he doesn't like, the reviews can be downright harsh:

> When you fast do not put on a gloomy look as the hypocrites do; they pull long faces to let people know they are fasting. I tell you, they have had their reward. But when you fast, put oil on your head and wash your face so that no one will know you are fasting except your Father who sees all that is done in secret; and your Father, who sees all that is done, will reward you (Matthew 6:16-18).

This is not meant to make us neurotic about hiding it from everybody when we're going without food. It is simply making us aware that if we aim our actions at pleasing people and impressing them, this is all the benefit we can expect: the esteem of those around us. The real work of prayer and fasting is interior. It is not the exterior actions that others can observe which produce vitality, but the dialogue of heart with heart, the contact of Spirit with spirit.

In practice this may mean that you go out of the office at noontime and take a walk or spend a quiet half hour in a nearby church, if staying at your desk and working right through is going to make your colleague or secretary start asking questions. And if someone should notice that you're not eating in spite of your efforts not to make an issue out of it, a simple "I'll be eating later, my schedule's a little different today' or an "I'm feeling fine as I am right now" kind of statement suffices. The point is simply not to flaunt it. If you find yourself going through machinations and subterfuge to "cover-up," chances are more energy is going into that than into a focusing of your heart upon God.

Expect Something to Happen

Trying to say just what I mean here is a bit tricky because the idea could so easily be conveyed that fasting puts God into a hammerlock or full-nelson wrestling hold to which he *has* to respond. I don't mean that at all. What I'm trying to get at here is that wonderful sense of personalness that the men and women of the Old Testament had with God. They *really believed* God is Someone who

81

is closer to us than the space between bodies hugging, more interested in us than a mother caring for her sick daughter, more ready to give to us than a husband assisting his wife during the act of childbirth. And out of this sense, that he is *here*, falling over himself to give us what we need, they went to him with a statement of how badly they *wanted*. They fully expected a response of one sort or another because they didn't know of anybody among those who loved them who could possibly be unresponsive in the face of such a laying-bare of the heart.

My dad told me once that he used to ride on his bicycle around the block where my mother lived just hoping to get a glimpse of her through the window. Israel's sense of God's love for her must have been like what my mother felt. She knew he was out there, circling, watching, hoping. And when she went to the window or came outside, she fully expected that he would act as if he knew her, and he would listen to her concerns with full attention, and that he would make a loving response.

That's what I mean by "expecting something to happen." Fasting is sending God a message. He's very good about answering his mail.

Some Preliminary Questions

As important as these kinds of reflections are for helping us enter into fasting as a religious act, we are still children of a scientific, technological, health-conscious age. We have seen too many hoaxes perpetrated in the name of religion, too many people taken advantage of, too many people get really "high" on something only to drop it later in disillusionment. We cannot, nor should we, just gloss over some of the very real and honest questions that lurk in the back of our minds. We feel a need to go forward slowly, cautiously, checking fasting out from every angle before we invest in it.

If someone you know wanted to talk seriously with you about something that she really believed in,you would listen and ask questions. The questioning response is completely natural and normal, and no question, when flowing from an honest spirit of inquiry, is off-limits or irrelevant. If your acquaintance thought it would be a good idea for you to invest some of your own time and energy into what she is committed to, your questions would probably be all the more far-ranging and thorough.

Well, consider me an acquaintance. Chances are you know more about how I think at this point than you do about a lot of other people you consider your acquaintances. Since we don't have the advantage of a face-to-face dialogue, I've tried to anticipate what some of your questions might be about fasting:

Is it safe? "Me fast? Are you serious? I don't want to die!" If we're honest with ourselves, we may recognize at least a tinge of that reaction in our own response to the proposal of fasting. At the bottom of the reaction seems to be a confusion between fasting and starvation. But they are two different concepts.

Fasting is a positive, freely chosen action that bestows a number of benefits. Starving, in contrast, is usually an involuntary wasting away through the prolonged unavailability of food or inadequate amounts of food.

The word "fast" derives from *faestan* (Old English: to abstain). The abstention is voluntary and undertaken for good effects. It is life-enhancing. The word "starvation" comes from the Old English *sterofan*, a derivation of the Teutonic verb *sterben*, which means "to die."

When we fast, we in effect decide that we are going to take our nourishment from the "reserves" we have been storing up in good supply. Starvation begins when the "storage shelves" have been emptied, when the body has consumed its spare resources, craves food, and continues to be deprived.

When the body is not receiving the needed nutrition via new incoming food, particularly proteins and fats, it will burn and digest its own tissues by the process of autolysis or self-digestion. The body, however, does not perform this process of autolysis indiscriminately. In its wisdom, the body will first decompose and burn those cells and tissues which are diseased, aged, damaged, or dead and this is where fasting earns the reputation of being a curative and rejuvenative therapy. Simply stated, the body feeds itself on the most impure and inferior materials, such as dead cells and morbid accumulations and fat deposits. It is for this reason that Dr. Otto Buchinger, one of the greatest authorities on fasting in the world, calls fasting a "refuse disposal, a burning of rubbish." Rest assured, however, that the essential tissues and vital organs, the glands, the nervous system and the brain are not damaged or digested in fasting.

At the same time that these old cells and diseased tissues are decomposed and burned, the building of new, healthy cells is expedited. Fasting speeds up the elimination of dead and dying cells, as well as accelerates the building of new cells. At the same time, the toxic waste products that interfere with the nourishment of the cells are effectively eliminated and the normal metabolic rate and cell oxygenation are restored.

It is essential to clear up the misconception that fasting is the same as starvation. They represent entirely different periods in the process of abstaining from food. The fasting stage continues so long as the body supports itself on the stored reserves within its tissues. Starvation begins when abstinence is carried beyond the time when these stored reserves are used up or have dropped to a dangerously low level.

It takes a very long fast to cross the line into starvation. The body has some finely tuned warning systems that give the signal when it is time to break fast. That time does not usually occur, according to Dr. Cott, until at least the twenty-fifth day, which is far, far beyond in length the kinds of fasts we'll be talking about in this book.

Fasting *is* safe for almost everybody. (Those who are responsible for the "almost" in that sentence will be specified in the next question.)

Unfortunately, we live in a society that practically equates "three squares a day" with the preservation of life itself. We live with a mistaken notion: that to miss a meal or two would be hazardous to our health and well-being. We don't, however, have as grave a problem with overeating. That, we rationalize, allows us to store up reserves for that "emergency situation" when we may have to miss a meal.

What we have yet to understand is that the body tolerates a fast far better than a feast. It has ample resources to nourish itself for surprisingly long periods of time. The process of nutrition continues to take place from the body's "cupboard," and as far as the organs that benefit know, food is still being eaten.

As Susan Smith Jones notes in *Runner's World*, the fast exerts a normalizing, stabilizing and rejuvenative effect on all the vital physiological, nervous and mental functions. The nervous system is rejuvenated, mental powers are improved, glandular chemistry and hormonal secretions are stimulated and increased, and the biochemical and mineral balance of the tissue is normalized.

Should I See a Doctor? Most people, it seems, don't consult a doctor before starting a fast, anymore than they do before starting a diet. But what have you got to lose? If you have a check-up before you fast, you're on the safe side. It will reveal if you have any of the following conditions listed by Dr. Cott, any one of which will rule fasting out in your case:

Heart diseases, especially a predisposition to thrombosis
Tumors
Bleeding ulcers
Cancer
Blood diseases
Active pulmonary diseases
Diabetes
Gout
Liver diseases
Kidney diseases
Cerebral diseases
Recent myocardial infarction

Pregnant women and women who have just given birth should not fast. If you are a "golden ager," make sure you have the blessings of your doctor. If you are very thin, you should not fast for more than a couple of days every few months. A person who has been taking drugs over a long period should fast only under medical supervision.

If you find yourself in any of the above conditions, it simply remains to you in that case to take a broader approach to fasting than to see it just in terms of abstention from *food*. There are many things that fog our lenses and make it difficult for us to keep our hearts clearly focused upon what is truly central and important in our lives. The spirit of fasting, i.e., what it seeks to do, can be present just as well in abstaining from watching T.V., from listening to the stereo or radio, or from using the telephone, especially when the time those activities would normally fill is given to something nurturing for our life in the Spirit (keeping a journal, reading a good book, or meditating).

Should I Alter My Routine of Activity When I Fast? No, there's no reason to. The only difference is that you don't eat. Every healthy person who observes a day of fast with any kind of regularity should be able to go about normal social and work routines. In other words, "business as usual." There is no psychological and physiological reason for cutting back on activity. Fasting for a short period is perfectly compatible with a full work load and an active participation in play. You will instinctively know if you have to cut back a bit; you're body will tell you if you're overdoing it. Contrary to your

85

expectation, as wastes and excesses and poisons are eliminated from the body, you may feel *more* energy and more vigor than when you were eating three substantial meals a day.

What About Exercise? Your body needs a lot of assistance in the form of fresh air, increased circulation and exercise in order to accomplish a thorough cleansing of the blood and tissues to effectively regenerate and revitalize all the bodily functions. So, by all means stay active. Don't think that your body isn't capable of sustaining any energy output. During a fast of two or even three days, there's no reason why you can't play golf or bowl or go cycling—if that is your normal form of exercise. In a three-day retreat that I made recently, while fasting for the three days, I went cross-country skiing for two hours the first day and jogged three or four miles the second and third day. I felt fine. Obviously everyone has a different tolerance to activity. Dr. Cott, consciously taking a cautious line for his general audience, draws the line at something as strenuous and sustained as long-distance jogging because of the continuously intensive nature of the activity. But a long, brisk walk of a couple of hours would be great. If you happen to be feeling tired and weak, well then by all means listen to that and rest and sleep as much as you can.

In *Fasting As a Way of Life*, Cott explodes the myth that anybody engaging in strenuous exercise must, in order to turn in a peak performance, stoke up before participating. It may come as revolutionary to those raised on the sacred dictum of "a steak before the game" to know that many professional athletes are foregoing food before competition. The American College of Sports Medicine, based in Madison, Wisconsin, has promulgated the opinion that the traditional pregame meal is not essential. "In fact, we have observed over many years that some of the truly great athletes ate absolutely nothing before competition."

Before an event, the traditional thinking has gone, athletes had to stock up on huge steaks, mounds of scrambled eggs, pitchers of milk, and platters of toast and honey. It is now grasped by many coaches that the energy needed to digest such a meal is deflected from performance. The food acts as an extra load, contributes to fatigue, and is still lodged in the stomach after the event is over. The body does not depend on food consumed just *before* or *during* heightened activity. It performs with the reserves it has accumulated over a period of time. Hence, "steak on game day" is a drag, not a lift. Its protein doesn't convert into energy quickly enough to be helpful. Of all the nutrients, protein takes the most time to digest. It also overburdens the elimination system at a time when it is already overworked with heavy perspiring.

Food and Fitness Magazine wrote of candy bars and other boosters: "The entire 'quick energy' myth is a giant rip-off invented by the very industry that led you to eat things that make you feel sluggish in the first place." Whereas a chocolate bar will give a quick lift for a very short time, it will then drop you like a weight-lifter does his barbells.

"I have discovered no reason," Cott says, "why the healthy person who is fasting for a few days shouldn't continue with the type of exercise to which he or she is accustomed. Failure to exercise, in fact, brings on fatigue. Exercise slows down the activity of the pancreas and this prevents a lowering of the sugar level and avoids fatigue."

In all of the above, it is mature, fully developed people who exercise regularly that are being talked about—not growing gradeschool or high-school youngsters. Young people during their growth period should never fast except in a medically controlled situation.

Are There Actually any Good Physical Effects that Can Be Relied Upon? Yes, and we'll go into them more thoroughly in Chapter 6 on Fasting and Fitness when we discuss just how fasting works, but for now, briefly: Fasting brings a welcome physiological rest for the digestive tract and the central nervous system. It normalizes metabolism. Normally, in addition to digesting food, which is its biggest job, the body works to eliminate wastes, fight diseases, ward off sickness, replenish worn-out cells, and nourish the blood. When it is relieved of its biggest job, the digestion of food, the system can catch up on some of its "backwork" in those other areas. Since it has more energy to bring to body-processes like warding-off sickness and nourishing the blood, both of which leave us feeling much better, the physical benefits of fasting are obvious.

Should I Continue with Vitamins and Minerals? As regards vitamins, minerals, and other food supplements, some say "discontinue," others "go ahead and keep on taking them if you want to." Dr. Stuart Hill, member of the Science Council of Canada, makes the point that taking vitamins can lead to problems because vitamins contain other substances than the specific vitamins. These substances, e.g., the corn filler or covering of many vitamins, may trigger allergic reactions to food substances, which allergic reactions are normally masked by other foods. Hence the recommendation that one should not take vitamins, medication of pills or any other kind without a doctor's approval. Besides that, keep warm, get plenty of fresh air, avoid hot baths and saunas, and make tobacco and alcohol part of what you're fasting from; if you're going to let your body clean house, it doesn't make much sense to sweep some of the toxins out the back door and bring more in the front door.

What about weight loss? One usually loses in a one- to three-day fast about one to two pounds of weight a day, mainly in fat tissue. Muscle, bone, blood and viscera lose proportionately much less of their total substance, and nerve tissue loses no weight. This is easily gained back after the fast, if it is part of your "ideal" weight. We return to what should be our normal weight very easily, if the fast has brought us below that. Fasting does bring us to that optimal weight level.

Should Children Fast? Dr. Bill Dietz, a nutritionist at the MIT Clinical Research Center and at Children's Hospital in Boston, says negative nitrogen balance can set in quickly if young children abstain from all food. He suggests they participate in a fast by eating small balanced meals, giving up junk food, meat, or something else that helps them feel they are sharing in the family fasting experience.

A Holistic Approach

A final; important "foreword" before we get to "the how" of fasting. When we begin to consider the "nuts 'n bolts" of fasting—the why's, the how's, the when's—there will be temptation to label different reasons, e.g., that's a "spiritual" reason, or that's a "physical" reason.

Resist that temptation. The more we let ourselves apply labels, the longer we keep alive the old "man/woman is composed of body and soul" dichotomy, and the longer we ignore all that the various sciences have learned about the seamless unity of the human person who is an enfleshed spirit, an animated body. In view of this unity, the approach here is holistic, i.e., dealing with the human person as an embodied spirit.

In practice what that means is that we operate from the presumption that what is good for us physiologically is also good for us spiritually; what is good for us spiritually is also good for us physiologically. There's only one "I" to my being. You can discuss different aspects of me, but I have only one being, and in the end you're still just talking about *me.*

An example: our main objective is to rediscover the value of fasting as an act of faith, hope, and love, a religious act, directed toward God. As such we have talked about fasting in terms of a focus of the heart, as a behavior that clears away the thousand little things that accumulate and clutter the heart and mind. It's like removing the rust and corrosion from a car battery to enable the current to flow more freely. It renews our "contact" with God.

At the same time, there is also another dimension of myself that needs the clutter and excess removed—the physiological dimension of myself. It has accumulated a lot of mucus and toxins and drugs and chemicals that if unloaded would enable the vital current of life to flow through me much more freely.

The temptation is to label the former one as "spiritual" and the latter as "physical," the one as good for my "soul," and the other as good for my "body."

But it's all *me*. And, therefore, it's all related. It is with my *self*, my embodied spirit, that I respond to God. If my digestive system is weighted down, blocked, overloaded, lethargic, that's going to influence my heart-response to God as regards my experience of the goodness of life. If you feel awful for physiological reasons, God is not likely to get many overflowings of joy and praise from your mouth.

But if I feel that every physical thing is running smoothly, if I feel the energy is flowing, if I feel productive and useful to others and, well, *healthy!*—then, how much more easily prayer will come! How much more easily will God's Spirit find a receptive response in my heart to the idea of fasting as a focus of my heart upon my God. Fasting will flow as a prayer right out of my visceral experience of gratitude, of joy in being alive. My thanks will be looking for a place to explode, for Someone to receive what I feel in the depths of my being.

So let's not lick any labels. Leave them in the box where they belong. If fasting is doing something positive for myself under any of its aspects, it is bringing me that much closer to an experience of joy and gratitude. And once I'm on that path, the ambush by God is only a matter of time.

The How of Fasting

The best way to begin in fasting is to ease into it. Start just by giving up one meal. Then, some days later, or the following week, drop two meals. Then next time around, try a whole day with nothing but water. Gradually, the fast can be increased to two or three consecutive days. Fasts that exceed three to five days in length are beyond the scope of this book and should be undertaken with medical supervision, for reasons that will be set forth later in this chapter.

In order to avoid getting entangled in a new system of distinctions between fast, partial fast, fast and abstinence, etc., I am going to give one definition to what I mean by fast and from then on when I use the word there will be no ambiguity about what is being referred to.

Fasting = certain liquids only. What kinds of liquids? There are two schools of thought on the question. I'll present them both, and you can make your own decision as to which of them has more "going" for it. As you will see, it is not a question of one being bad and the other being good, but of two "goods," one perhaps being slightly better than the other.

Opinion A: The best, most effective, and safest way to fast is water fasting. Simple enough? Cool water, warm water, Perrier water, distilled water, tap water, water in an elegant goblet to make it look like the elixir of life that it is. Artificially colored, flavored, and sweetened drinks recall the memory of food to our tastebuds and arouse distracting hunger, and at the same time inhibit the purifying process that is going on in the digestive system.

Fasting means total abstention from caloric intake, which includes fruit and vegetable juices. Hence, only water is taken during a fast. Certain herbal teas and juices are sometimes used to promote elimination, as are various types of enemas and baths. However, taking foods, even vitamins, can lead to problems. Foods can trigger allergic reactions by creating nutritional imbalances that are corrected by the body robbing from itself.

The water one drinks should ideally be at room temperature, and bottled water is recommended if it is available. Most tap water contains chlorine and flourides, manufactured chemicals. At a time when one is interested in cleansing one's system, it makes sense not to ingest more chemicals.

Apart from the oxygen in the air we breathe, the most important ingredient for humans is water, which constitutes between one-half and three-quarters of the weight of every human. This percentage is higher in babies and young children than in adults, and in lean rather than obese individuals. The intracellular fluid—the water inside the individual cells—constitutes three-quarters of the total body water.

Although water generally is not thought of as a nutrient, it is absolutely essential to every bodily function. Every chemical change that occurs in the body takes place in the presence of water.

In addition, water is the basis of every body fluid—blood, lymph, digestive juices, bile, perspiration, urine, and feces. It acts like oil in an engine, lubricating and preventing friction between moving parts, and it regulates body temperature through evaporation from the lungs as the result of perspiration.

The primary use of water in our bodies involves kidney function, since it is the kidneys through which waste products are excreted. Once this task is completed, water is made available within the body for other purposes.

Opinion B: The best, most effective and safest way to fast is juice-fasting. According to Dr. Buchinger, fasting on fresh raw juices of fruits and vegetables, plus vegetable broths and herb teas results in much faster recovery from disease and more effective cleansing and rejuvenation of the tissues than does the traditional water fast. Dr. Ragnar Berg, a world-famous authority on nutrition and biochemistry, says:

> During fasting the body burns up and excretes huge amounts of accumulated wastes. We can help this cleansing process by drinking alkaline (having the property of soluble salt) juices instead of water while fasting. I have supervised many fasts and made extensive examinations and tests of fasting patients, and I am convinced that drinking alkali-forming fruit and vegetable juices, instead of water, during the fasting will increase the healing effect of fasting. Elimination of uric acid and other inorganic acids will be accelerated. And the sugars in juices will strengthen the heart. . . . .Juice fasting is, therefore, the best form of fasting.

Vitamins, minerals, enzymes, trace elements and fresh, raw vegetable juices are extremely beneficial in normalizing all body processes. They supply needed elements for the body's own healing activity and cell regeneration and expedite the recovery. These juices require no digestion and are easily assimilated directly into the blood-stream. They do not disrupt the healing and rejuvenating process of autolysis, or "refuse disposal."

Since all fruits and vegetables are plants (herbs), they possess specific medicinal properties. Fresh juices are also medicinal (healing) in their action and can be used to advantage in therapeutic fasting. The juices should be as fresh as possible; in the best of all ideal worlds, juiced at home right before drinking. The next best thing: buy fresh raw juices at your local health-food store. A couple of *caveats*: avoid juices that have pulp in them, and don't mix fruit and vegetable juices together (the mixture of the two may not sit well with your stomach). Dilute the sweeter juices such as orange, carrot, and apple 50/50 with water to prevent shocking the finely balanced blood glucose system and its concomitant organ, the pancreas. The total juice or broth volume will generally be between 1½ pints and 1½ quarts per day, though some speak of taking up to a gallon of juices if they have been exercising strenuously. This juice volume is in addition to the recommended six to eight daily glasses of water, whether one is fasting or not, and, while fasting, even if it is a juice fast.

Adults generally lose six percent of body water per day; infants, about fifteen percent. The amount of water loss is affected by physical activity, body and environmental temperatures, humidity and wind velocity. A person performing hard physical labor in a hot, dry climate can lose about twelve quarts of water in perspiration alone. On the other hand, a deskbound worker who lives in a temperate climate may lose little more than a quart a day.

Water lost from the body can be replaced in a number of ways. The most obvious is by drinking, and an intake of six to eight glasses a day is desirable. All of this does not have to be in the form of water, but may include other beverages as well— fruit drinks, soft drinks, tea or coffee, and soups.

Additional sources of water are the solid foods we eat. Even dry cereals are from 8 to 20 percent water, meat contains from 40 to 75 percent water and fruits and vegetables from 75 to 90 percent.

Under normal circumstances, it is not very likely that an individual will ingest too much water. However, a person who is unusually thirsty or suddenly starts passing a great deal of urine should see a physician, since these may be symptoms of diabetes. Conversely, a swelling of parts of the body as a result of water retention also is a very strong indication of the need for medical attention.

When a person is subjected to extreme deprivation, it can result in death. A 10 percent loss of water constitutes a dangerous situation, while a 20 percent loss would be fatal.

It is best, at any time, not to drink water that is too cold. If you don't seem to be eliminating as much water as you're taking in and wonder where it's going, probably right out through your pores in the most dynamic organ of the elimination network.

Why these certain liquids only? Because we are seeking to quiet the self, in all ways, so that it can hear and be more attentive to him who is present to it and focus more upon this Presence. And drinks like black coffee and nonherbal teas stimulate the central nervous system at a time when we are trying to give the self a rest, a space and time for focus upon more internal realities.

When we drink only water or alkaline juices during a fast the human mechanism cleanses itself, the same as when we wring out a dirty sponge. The dirt in this case is toxins and drugs that have been passing around in our circulatory system trying to become so thoroughly dissolved that they can pass through the fine structure of the body's "physiological sieve," the kidneys. These certain liquids are a faster's best friends since they facilitate the flushing out of waste materials that keep our "self" running at low-level performance, feeling sluggish, and not very much in the mood to give God joyful praise for the gift of life and health. Each of our two kidneys has a million efficient filters, and when the body is fasting, the kidneys step up their work of detoxification. All the energy that is not being used up in the laborious task of mastication, digestion, metabolism, and elimination is turning its attention toward renewing our "self."

Arnold de Vries, in his book *Therapeutic Fasting*, writes that during fasting the eliminative and cleansing capacity of the eliminative organs—lungs, liver, kidneys, and the skin—is greatly increased and the masses of accumulated wastes and toxins are quickly expelled. He reports that during fasting the concentration of toxins in the urine can be ten times higher than normal. This is because the alimentary canal, liver and kidneys are relieved of the usual burden of digesting foods and eliminating wastes and toxins, such as uric acid and purines, from the tissues. Some of the normal symptoms that this cleansing process is taking place are offensive breath, dark urine, skin eruptions, excessive perspiration, and elimination of mucus through the nose and air passages.

Side-Effects You're Likely to Feel and What They Mean

Eating has become such an important part of our lives that when we deprive ourselves of food and begin a fast, we may experience one or more mental and physical reactions. Headaches. Nausea. Dizziness. Gnawing in the stomach. Coating on the tongue. Bad Breath. Restless sleep. These are the side-effects that have given fasting a bad name and made it very unpopular. But if we take the trouble to remove their masks, we'll find that they're not so bad after all. As a matter of fact, they're blessings in disguise. Signs of healing. A step on the way to feeling really well, both mentally and physically.

The good news is that they're transitory. They are indications that the body is ridding itself of waste materials. And the best news is that some people won't experience these unpleasantnesses or discomforts at all, even though the purification is going on. The faster's attitude has been known to make a big difference, e.g., the people who approach it positively, putting their apprehensions and fears behind as inappropriate, have the better record. But if you run into any of those blessings in disguise, here's how to respond to them:

Gnawing in the stomach: it's not a genuine hunger pang (in the sense that your body doesn't need the food), nor a distress signal. It's just the alimentary tract accommodating itself to a reduced work load. How to deal with it? Drink water more frequently—a glass of water can satisfy what feels like a ravenous appetite.

Coating on the tongue: The tongue is a mirror that reflects the amount of waste matter being eliminated. Normally, we associate bad smells with the processes of elimination. That explains why we may have bad breath: the tongue is part of the elimination system. Rinse your mouth with warm water, and gently brush your tongue with a soft toothbrush; then move on to your teeth. If your taste buds are sleeping nicely from lack of stimulation, and if you don't want to risk waking them, leave the caps on your flavored toothpaste and mouthwashes (though some would make the good point that charity to those you're working closely with demands using them!).

Tiredness, weakness, restless sleep, headache: what's happening is that when you fast, the waste in your body is being loosened and sent into the circulation system to be discarded. When this is going on you feel miserable. But once the waste is discarded, you begin to feel much better. As you fast, conditions change from day to day. If and when you encounter any of these signs, just bite the bullet and tough it out. All things pass, as they say, especially bodily waste if you give your body-person a chance to clean house. As you cleanse, you are going to feel stronger and it will have been well worth it. It seems a bit ironic, but it's the way it works: a seemingly healthy person has to pass first of all through a condition of sickness (cleansing), a kind of intermediate stage of illness, to get to a higher level of health. This is why people on prolonged fasts feel better and stronger on the tenth day of the fast than the second. The unobstructed blood circulation can now produce increased vitality. In the final chapter we will observe more closely the claims people make after fasting: my mind is more alert, I have better sex, my hair is growing again, I'm sleeping better, I don't have indigestion any more, and so on. The clinical reason given for why all these things can actually happen is that after the elimination of waste and poisonous materials with which the tissues and intestinal tract have been clogged up for years, normal bodily functioning can take place once again.

The "How Long" of Fasting

This is basically a question to be discerned in prayer. Anything we do to deepen the communion with our God is done only at the initiative of the Holy Spirit working in our hearts. It is the Spirit who gives the idea, the Spirit who inclines us to respond favorably to the idea, and the Spirit who urges us to move from idea to action. Without the Spirit enabling it, we can't even think about God. So the question of "how long should I fast?" is a question to be resolved in the depths of your heart where the Spirit dwells in the temple of your self. Related considerations will be your situation in life, the particular "why" (if there is one) of a fast at this time, and the circumstances of your workload.

I will provide here some helpful information for fasts of basically two durations: twenty-four to thirty-six hours, and three to five days.

Twenty-four to thirty-six-hour fast. In the case of a thirty-six-hour fast, going from dinner on Monday, say, to breakfast on Wednesday has the advantage of spanning two nights during which time the fast can be cleaning the temple of your embodied spirit with the full brunt of its energy because there's no other activity going on for which energy is needed. The twenty-four-hour fast may work best for some from lunch to lunch, and for others, from dinner to dinner. While you're sending God a message from your heart, you can give your digestive system an assist for the work it's trying to do by putting a third of a teaspoon of uncooked honey and a teaspoon of lemon juice in your water. These elements act as mucus and toxic dissolvers so that the poisons can be flushed out more easily. If you have never fasted before, work from skipping one meal to two meals up to a twenty-four-hour fast. After some regularity with this, you will have gained some experience and a stronger belief in fasting. You will have prepared yourself for a longer fast, if that is what the Spirit leads you to.

Three to five-day fast. A fast of three days or more should be conducted under conditions that are ideal to rest and quiet. You should be able to rest if you're feeling the effects of the poisons passing out of your body. During a fast of this duration it is quite possible that you could feel uncomfortable, so you should have the freedom to go to your room and lie down and relax there. Since the deepest motive for what you are doing relates to your life before God, use that time for reflection, prayer, or just being still and knowing that he is God and you are creature. Leave the books closed, the television and radio off, and cancel your social calendar for the evening. The ideal time and place for a fast like this is a retreat where you're already relieved from your work responsibilities, don't have anything or anybody else scheduled, and the stereo and T.V. aren't what you had in mind anyway when you came away to this place. You can sleep in the morning, take walks and naps as you feel inclined, and in general let your physical energy be used for detoxification and internal cleansing. This kind of unpressured space is also the time when God very often takes advantage of our heart's quietness and tranquillity to speak to us about his dream for us, what he would like us to do, how he would like us to develop and use our talents and abilities. A combination fasting/retreat experience like this can be totally rejuvenating for the whole person.

Hunger, amazingly, disappears during a fast that extends beyond a couple days. It may seem incredible that you can completely give up eating and not feel hungry, but it's true. The reason is that as long as you are eating anything at all, the palate is in a state of stimulation—savoring the last meal, anticipating the next one. When nothing is consumed, there is no "memory" of food to titillate the taste buds. Any hunger pangs are mild and superficial. *The Journal of the American Medical Association* noted, in reporting this phenomenon, that by contrast, people on diets often report feeling constantly hungry. Strange as it seems, the indication

is that it's easier to sacrifice food altogether than to try to stick to a diet low in calories. When you eat nothing at all, the body steps up its production of ketones, which are broken-down products of fatty acids. They are released into the bloodstream, and as they increase in quantity they suppress the appetite. This accounts for why a person who is fasting from two five days feels that he or she could continue the fast without discomfort and is breaking it through *choice* and not a sense of famished hunger. Along with this there is a feeling of breathing easier, greater freedom of movement (e.g., Yoga postures), and the departure of that dragged-out feeling.

Since all the fasting researchers that I have been mentioning along the way express themselves in favor of the shorter, regular fast over the longer fasts more infrequently taken, I do not feel it would be responsible for me to deal with anything beyond three to five days, which for the researchers qualifies as a "short fast." One of the reasons they do not believe in long fasts of three and four weeks unless carefully supervised by an expert is that the average person is not only filled with toxic poisons from eating the wrong kinds of food, air pollution, water pollution, and various chemicals, but he or she also has a residue of many drugs that are stored deep in the organs of the body. It is better, they say, to try to remove these large amounts of toxic waste from the body by a weekly fast-day and an occasional three- or four-day fast along with a wholesome regular diet, than to try to clean the body with one long fast. With such intermittent fasts, the blood is gradually improved, regenerated, and can more easily tolerate the poisons and waste, and the person is able little by little to dissolve and eliminate disease deposits from the deepest tissues of the body—deposits that no other method of healing has ever discovered or can remove.

There was more genius in the bygone Christian practice of weekly fasting than we realized. The world of science is now coming forward and telling us that such a practice makes a great deal of sense not only for the health of our relationship with God, but for the health of ourselves too! When all the data is in from different sectors of our human experience, the reasons for a return (with clearer understanding this time) to the practice of a weekly fast day are all the more compelling.

How to Come Off the Fast

Gandhi once said that perhaps more caution and more restraint are necessary in breaking a fast than in keeping it. Breaking a fast is a very important and significant phase of the fasting process. The beneficial physiological effects can be quickly undone if the fast is incorrectly broken. In other words: begin with little and take even that slowly. Eating too much too fast can lead to digestive upset and general disorder. Some things to keep in mind:

—For three days of fasting, include one day as a transition day. After a two-day fast, figure on two transitional meals; after a one-day fast, one transitional meal. Transitional meals consist of natural foods void of overly processed ingredients such as white sugar, white flour, and preservatives, e.g., a piece of fruit and/or fresh vegetable soup with juice or herb tea.

—The first meal after the fast should be designed to have a cleansing laxative effect, rather than for its nourishment value. The first food that reaches your taste buds should be along the lines of a raw variety vegetable salad with a base of grated carrots and grated cabbage. Lemon juice makes a good dressing. The effect of this salad will be that of a big broom moving right through your thirty feet of intestines. It will give the muscles along the gastointestinal tract something to work with, too. Follow this salad with cooked vegetables, i.e., stewed tomatoes, spinach, squash, celery, or string beans. You'll find that a little bit of food can seem like a great sufficiency. Continue to drink lots of water. Eat slowly and chew carefully.

—Depending on how long your fast has been, wait a corresponding amount of time before getting into foodstuffs like meat, milk, cheese, butter, fish, nuts and seeds. Do not eat any more than you desire. There's no need to compensate for all the food that wasn't eaten because appetite doesn't accumulate like that. And just because you're eating is no guarantee that you're going immediately to feel a surge of energy. It takes time for the body to adjust from a detoxicating program to an eating. Avoid turning around and overburdening your digestive system just after giving it a rest.

The When of Fasting

We need to rediscover fasting as an appropriate behavior for Christian *life*. Not just for Ash Wednesday or Good Friday or even the whole of Lent. But for Christian LIFE.

The greatest commandment, Jesus said, is to love the Lord your God with your whole heart, your whole soul, and with all your strength. That's the fundamental rationale we have been considering for fasting: to place God more at the center of our lives, to better focus our consciousness upon him with our whole enfleshed spirit. If fasting helps us respond to the greatest commandment there is, can we afford to lose it or to confine it to just a certain season?

And now that we know how it helps us care for the self God has given us, the second greatest commandment takes on new meaning: "You shall love your neighbor *as your self*" (emphasis mine). Would we want our neighbor to be poisoned, living in an unhealthy environment, functioning at half of his or her potential, experiencing only a fraction of the joy and vitality that God meant us all to know? Of course not! All our social-action programs are aimed at providing "our neighbor" with what is needed for a truly and fully human existence.

If that's what I want for my neighbor and what I'm obliged to seek for him or her, the same measure is to be applied to myself. Fasting becomes social action carried out upon myself!

If God lived in a temple down the street, and I were the caretaker, I'm sure I wouldn't allow it to be strewn and littered with waste and garbage. I'd see that as a clear sign of disrespect to the One who is present. Now, as I apply that to myself as a temple in whom the Trinity dwells, what's the difference?

For all of these reasons, I suggest a re-embracing of our earlier Christian practice of a fast day each week. Furthermore, I think the earlier custom of observing the Ember Days has a lot to recommend it. They were originally Christian replacements for seasonal festivals of agrarian cults. They were observances of penance, thanksgiving, and petition for divine blessing on the various seasons. As such they were observed four times a year. A weekly fast day, coupled with a three-day fast four times a year, once in each season of Advent, Lent, Pentecost, and thanksgiving for the harvest, would restore fasting as a behavior for Christian *life*.

We would, of course, have to choose to do something like this *freely* because of the value we see in it. There can be no going back to those laws which say we *have* to do it. They will just make us lose the spirit of it all over again. With this approach, our fasting would have to flow out of our prayer, our sense of the season, our awareness of what's going on in the life of the Lord as we relive it through the liturgical year. With this approach, our fasting would flow out of our own interior sense that *it's time*. Time to focus our hearts. To give special praise and thanks at this time of Christmas. To do penance. To make straight the way of the Lord in Lent. To pray in this Easter season to receive the Spirit of the Lord in a new Pentecost. To let our whole being overflow with gratitude, as do our harvest bins at the end of summer in autumn's golden days.

We have become too fractured, too insulated. We celebrate festival days without ever feeling the growing urge within us to celebrate because *it is time* to celebrate. The liturgical seasons were founded upon an agrarian calendar that was shaped according to what was going on in nature. Today, in our urban living, we have become so distanced from the rhythm of the land that it is more difficult for us to feel an instinctive harmony with an agrarian cycle. How can we bring the ebb and flow of the liturgical seasons and our lives back together again? How can we recapture the harmony and unity of it all? The body of our tradition is lying in pieces about us, and there is no breath in it.

Were we more in touch with what is going on in the world of nature about us, what is going on in the life of the church, what is going on within ourselves, we would fast at other times, too. Jesus tied the timing of when we fast to a question of appropriateness:

Can the children of the bridechamber fast while the bridegroom is with them? As long as they have the bridegroom with them, they cannot fast. But the days will come when the bridegroom will be taken away from them, then they will fast in those days (Mark 2:19, 20).

He linked fasting to the immediate circumstances, to felt needs. It was to be an honest reaction, one growing out of real life.

Fasting as an Honest Reaction to What's Going on in My Life

To my need for conversion. There are times when I know I need to turn again to the Lord with renewed fervor. Times when I need conversion. Times that deeper, more thorough self-examination and repentance may be required for me to find God in the way I need to find him. Repeated petition seems unavailing and direction is not forthcoming. I know that my prayer is distracted and half-hearted and falls back upon me in empty words. I am too full of myself to really settle down and wait for God. I am in a mood to be distracted.

100

Give me a movie and I'll go. What does the TV guide have to offer this week? Whom haven't I been out with for awhile? It is time to fast. Time to let God strip away what has piled up between us.

The Lord told us that if we judge ourselves, we will not need to be judged. Fasting is one means of pulling ourselves up short before God and letting him search our hearts. As soon as we begin to feel cluttered and out of touch, we can turn to God and ask him to show us why this coolness between us is happening. David's prayer can become our own:

> Search me, O God, and know my heart;
> try me, and know my thoughts.
> See if there be any wicked ways in me,
> and lead me in the way everlasting

(Psalm 139:23,24)

Why wait until we are backed against the wall and seeking God as the only alternative? God is concerned with our focus because it determines our steering, our direction. And periodically, depending on the constellation of circumstances in our lives, it needs readjustment. He allows us to get into certain situations that will show us whether our hearts are set upon him or intent upon pleasing ourselves. Is God central, or are things? What matters most to us?

To grief and distress. Another time in my life when I may turn to fasting as an honest reaction is in grief, distress, and mourning. After he had been knocked off his horse on the road to Damascus, Paul fasted for three days, waiting in total blindness for further instructions from the Lord. It must have been a time of complete upheaval and reversal of life purposes for him. His anxiety must have been extreme. In the Old Testament, Ezra was so disturbed by the sin of his countrymen that he found no better way to express the intensity of his grief and sorrow than this: "He ate no bread and drank no water, for her mourned their transgression . . . " (Ezra 10:6). David's fasting, too, was an honest reaction to the death of Saul and of Jonathan. He could not desire food while the emotions of shock and loss swept over him, so he set aside time for his reactions. He did not try to go on with business as usual, masking his feelings:

> Then David took hold on his clothes and rent them; and . . .
> mourned and wept and fasted . . . for Saul, and for Jonathan his

101

son, and for the people of the Lord, and for the house of Israel, because they were fallen by the sword

(2 Samuel 1:11,12).

To fatigue. The recognition that I need a rest is another moment in the year when fasting is an honest reaction. "Come to me, all you who are heavy burdened, and I will give you rest . . . learn of me and you will find rest for your souls." I am worn out. I am tired of the sound of my own voice. When someone comes to the door or the phone rings, it feels like an imposition. My mind keeps straying as I am listening to this person. Somebody calls a meeting and my first thought is, "How long will it last?" I don't even want to know what is in my heart because I don't have the energy to deal with it. I just saw my good friend and it didn't feel special to me to see him at all. I feel driven. I can't laugh at the mess on my desk; I resent it.

I need time to get in touch with myself and to pour out my heart to God. Rest is essential. Fasting makes it a total rest, for *all* of me. In the Mosaic Law, a special day was set aside in which no work was to be done and the people were to fast. The reason? To free the people from daily cares and family responsibilities so that they could deal with their inner life. What a great idea!

To travel. When I moved to Canada a couple of years ago, I noticed that people didn't speak of vacations but referred instead to "holiday." It's a British influence, for the old English word for "rest day" was "holiday"—hearkening back to a time when rest time was holy time, a holy day. Oftentimes, unfortunately, when we come to that extended rest time in the year called "vacation" or "holiday," we so plan, control, and package it that it's finished before beginning, dead before having a chance to live. We trek through a predetermined scene that only amounts to a life-sized version of pictures we looked at even before we left home. Returning from such a time away, there is an experience of relief: we made it through that potentially unpredictable time without a scratch. We're back, just as we left. No window flew open with a view of God-knows-what unsettling unpredicted thing. Keeping that window closed was tense and complicated. But we did it. And we're home safe.

Sometimes it can be a wonderful experience to trust that life is basically confident and gracious at its heart and to enter into life's persn had more time than a single holiday, a frequent way of stretching it out was by making a pilgrimage. Anagarika Govinda, a German-born Buddhist who is now a very old man in the United States, describes the meaning of pilgrimage:

102

A pilgrimage distinguishes itself from an ordinary journey by the fact that it does not follow a laid-out plan or itinerary, that it does not pursue a fixed aim, or a limited purpose, but that it carries its meaning in itself, by relying on an inner urge which operates on two planes, physical and spiritual. It is a movement, not only in the outer, but equally in the inner space, a movement whose spontaneity is that of the nature of all life, i.e., a movement that always starts from an invisible inner core (*The Way of the White Clouds*).

When I approach my holiday in this spirit—whether it's just a day off or a three-week vacation—fasting often enters into it very spontaneously. I may be driving from one place to another and just decide to keep right on going without stopping to eat; or perhaps the plane arrival and departure times are out of "sync" with meal times; or I may be trying to decide what to take with me on a day hike or a bike tour, and the thought will come to me: "Why take anything at all?" If the time in front of me is planned out roughly rather than rigidly, if where I'm going and what I'll do amounts to no more than an expedient structure, a kind of loose net within which my sight will be on the little open spaces between the netting, tiny inspirations can suggest themselves along the way and find a fertile ground for response. When time away is approached in the spirit of pilgrimage, one enters into it flexibly, waiting on God, expecting unforeseen paths to present themselves. And through all one sees and does and feels, there is a kind of alertness to the Divine Presence beneath the surface, an openness that is gently expectant, willing to be caught up and pulled into the freshness of divine play.

As crazy as it may sound, fasting can be like that: a secret shared between oneself and God, an act of a free spirit, a lighthearted feeling of liberation as one flaunts the convention of eating and locates joy and interest elsewhere. The impulse to make a day in the middle of vacation a fast day can, if responded to with the spirit of a pilgrim, be a deeply enjoyable day that has a positive quality about it that is different from all the other days. And no wonder. It hearkens back to a time when a holiday was a holy time, a holy day.

To receiving the Eucharist. And as a final example of fasting as an honest reaction to realities in our lives, why don't we take another look at the Eucharistic fast and try to rediscover what that was all about? Fasting can be a good barometer of the range of our consciousness. When something or someone greater is coming my way, I'm willing to say "forget it" to eating. It seems to me that underneath the Eucharistic fast was the idea that God is more important to me than life itself, and I impress that truth upon myself and prepare myself to meet him by setting aside that which symbolizes life for me. And then I will receive as my food the Bread that comes down from heaven. Fasting has created a psychic space within, and now Christ comes to fill me with his hunger and his thirst. This expresses the meaning of the Eucharistic fast and the early church's fasting before Baptism or Ordination, before the dedication of a church or on the vigils of the great feasts commemorating the joys of our redemption. There is a sense of joy and anticipation at the coming of the Savior who brings more health and greater life.

Fasting is Christian when it is rooted in hope. When we reach the Kingdom of Heaven, hope is no longer needed, because he whom we have been hoping for is ours. When we are all sitting around the divine banquet table described in Isaiah 25-6, there can be no further fasting. But now, before the eternal banquet, fasting and hope are honest reactions. The joy comes from what has already been given (though not yet fully), and from the anticipation of what still awaits us, wonders the likes of which "eye has not seen, nor ear heard."

Glory be to the Father, and to the Son, and to the Holy Spirit, who leads us in a desire to fast, gives us the proper intention, and accompanies us as our Advocate, bringing us into a few-found integration with ourselves and deeper communion with our God.

5 *Fasting for Others In the "Era of Me"*

> *We are part of a large community in which
> wealth is an obligation, resources are a
> trust, and joint action is a necessity.*
>
> —Henry Kissinger

> *If history remembers America in a kindly
> light, it will not be because its politicians
> wanted it to be Number One — we were first in
> the number of bombs, cars, and can openers —
> but because we were the first nation in
> history to decide collectively to feed the
> hungry at a personal sacrifice. If we
> aren't remembered for that, all other
> glories will be forgotten.*
>
> —Coleman McCarthy

> *Here were decent godless people;
> their only monument the asphalt road
> and a thousand lost golf balls.*
>
> —T. S. Eliot

"Many others are stretched out on the carpet all around her; some 249 other souls, in fact. They're all strewn across the floor of the banquet hall with their eyes closed, just as she is . . . concentrating on things that sound serious and deep when you talk about them. And how they had talked about them! They had all marched right up to the microphone and 'shared,' as the trainer called it. What did they want to eliminate from their lives? Why, they took their fingers right off the old repress button and told the whole room. My husband! My wife! My homosexuality! My inability to communicate, my self-hatred, self-destructiveness, craven fears, pulling weaknesses, primordial horrors, premature ejaculation, impotence, frigidity, rigidity, subservience, laziness, alcoholism, major vices, minor vices, grim habits, twisted psyches, tortured souls — and then it had been her turn, and she had said, 'Hemorrhoids!' "

So wrote Tom Wolfe in *New York* magazine, describing how the old alchemical dream of changing base metals into gold has changed: the new alchemical dream is changing one's personality—remaking, remodeling, elevating, and polishing one's very *self* . . . and observing, studying, and doting on it.

By the late 1960's North America was experiencing affluence on an unprecedented scale, bringing with it more leisure time, better education, a greater awareness of life's possibilities, higher expectations, and a rapid social mobility that was tearing apart the established webs of community and extended family. At the same time, there was a decline in the influence of religion, a decline in respect for all forms of authority, and a greater freedom of personal conduct than ever before. Many people had no idea of what to do with that freedom. The common man was getting quite interested in "realizing his potential as a human being" and he grabbed his money and ran, moving from the modest hope of living without fear to the grand need for existential purpose.

The latest psychotherapeutic breakthrough was therapy for the normal (now that there was the free time and surplus income, why should only the aristocratic intellectuals and artists be able to indulge in the luxury of dwelling upon their conduct and personality?). Therapy for the purpose of growth rather than cure. Therapy for normal, everyday people who say and do all the right things and get on well at their jobs but who just happen to want to grow, to get more out of their lives, to discover their inner selves, to be in better touch with themselves, making themselves more self-actualized, self-directed, self-assertive, self-fulfilled. Suddenly, masses of people were asking themselves questions that just twenty years ago would have been inconceivable. Questions like: "Who am I?" and "What should I be doing with my life?" and "How can I be happier?"

Twenty years before, the great majority of people were simply too busy earning a living to worry about such matters. And for those who did manage to snatch a few moments of existential agonizing, there were plenty of still-satisfactory traditional answers. You were a mother, a father, an insurance salesman, a teacher, a nurse. You should be using your life to serve others and your God, love your neighbor and raise your family. Could anything else possibly make you happier?

106

But "every age develops its own peculiar forms of pathology, which express in exaggerated form its underlying character," says social critic Christopher Lasch. He and others have said that ours is an age of narcissism (recalling the beautiful youth of Greek legend who fell in love with his reflection in a pool and pined away in rapture over it). As evidence of a growing narcissism in the national character, observers see: the preoccupation with self and the decline of interest in public life and social goals; the proliferation of therapies (Transactional Analysis, Primal Scream, Bioenergetics, Psychocybernetics, Rolfing, Sensitivity Training, Nude Marathon, Silva Mind Control, EST Scientology, Arica and Synanon) that declare we should be our own best friends and look out, above all, for "No. 1"; and the tendency to eschew marriage and childrearing in favor of remaining single, "living together," or living alone.

For those who are already married, there are also new types of therapy that are popular forms, currently, of "let's talk about me." Through group therapy, marriage counselling and other forms of psychological consultation, married couples can now enjoy that same "me" euphoria that the very rich have enjoyed for years in psychoanalysis. The cost of the new "me" sessions is only ten dollars to thirty dollars an hour, whereas psychoanalysis runs from fifty to one hundred twenty-five dollars.

A phenomenon even more recent than the new therapies, though now declining, is disco. When it first rose to ascendancy, many were already predicting that it would die within a year or two. That was several years ago, and the disco craze has danced on the tombs of its early nay-saying critics. In an article in the Montreal *Gazette* several patrons of local discos were interviewed as to why discos are so popular:

"It's an attention-grabber," says Mancini. "It fulfills a need people have of being looked at. For a minute you think you're Robert Redford."

Jennifer Martin, who has just taken a trip above the crowd on the chair-lift at Oz, (a local disco) observes: "You feel like a princess up there. You get down from the chair and people notice you and make a comment. You get a little glow inside for a while."

There are social scientists who see disco as the harbinger of a new age of hedonism. Others see it as a search for involvement

107

by people who are tired of spectator sports. Still others say it works against involvement: The mirrors, the volume of sound, the non-contact dancing contribute to what is essentially a narcissistic activity. Maryka de Orla, a 19-year-old university student, says everybody feels special on the dance floor.

"The lights are on you, and you're a star. A lot of people find that makes their night. Everybody I've talked to about it has said they like discos mainly because they can be Somebody."

A task force of the American Psychiatric Association preparing a new edition of the APA's diagnostic manual included in its draft a new syndrome called "narcissistic personality disorder" which it defines as combining an "exaggerated sense of self-importance" with a "lack of sustained positive regard" for others.

As we try to understand just what is happening in our society that is resulting in manifold forms of seemingly me-centered behavior, there is a need to keep the big picture in mind. How do these last ten to fifteen years represent a continuum, or a reaction, to what was going on in the previous twenty years? And what might we hope for next if where we are now is seen as just a corporate, elongated, developmental phase?

I think we must be open to the possibility that the Era of Me, for all its narcissistic behavior patterns, represents a movement *away from* the growing materialism that has marked our national life in the post-war boom. It may well be a movement within, symbolizing the failure of materialism to deliver genuine fulfillment. If it is such, it represents a progressive step in the quest of the human heart for integrity, peace, and inner joy. The quest is vitally human and unquestionably good. It is critical, however, that the search for fulfillment, which has now led within, not get stuck there. Once the journey within myself has served to show me that there is a self of irreplaceable worth and value there, it must move outward in affirmation, appreciation, respect, and celebration of the unique and infinitely valuable selves that others are, too. When that happens, we do not have people living within mirrored walls having a relationship with themselves. We have people capable of interacting for mutual growth, people who are sensitive to the delicate balance between assertiveness and surrender, people who have learned when to assert their own needs and wants and when to yield graciously to the wants and needs of the other. In that delicate balance, perhaps more than anywhere else, lies the secret of living together as members of the same human family.

Fasting as Ministry

As we try to reflect on fasting as a ministry *for others*, this broad-based retrenchment within (toward *me*) that is going on is the milieu in which we undertake the task of transcending ourselves and thinking of somebody else. The challenge is formidable because selfishness, ego-hunger, and moral blindness have asserted themselves in the larger culture through a pervasive and perhaps unconscious shift in values. In the moral definitions and judgments we make as individuals, they have been cast as enlightenment and psychic health. The world view emerging among us centers solely on the needs of the self and has individual survival as its main goal. It is a world view present not only in everything we say and do, but as an ambience, a feeling in the air, a general cast of perception and attitude: a retreat from the worlds of morality and history, an unembarrassed denial of human reciprocity and community.

In the previous chapter we considered fasting as *worship*, as an act of religion (*re-ligare*, Latin for re-tying), an act of tying or binding ourselves again to God, more tightly this time, humbly aware that we are creature and God is creator. We reflected on fasting as an act that recognizes the centrality of God's place in our lives, a faith-act that admits there is only One who can fill the deepest hungers of our being, a love-act that says, "You, the Giver of my life, are more important to me than even your gift of life which, synbolized by food, I set aside to focus my heart more clearly upon You."

In so doing, we are already transcending ourselves, already moving beyond Me as the center of the world. In this chapter, I want to take that self-transcending momentum further. It has been stated several times already that prayer, fasting, and works of charity are like three cogwheels, all working interdependently with one another. The time has come in our consideration of fasting to see where fasting and works of charity mesh.

St. Augustine sets the theme:

Don't believe that fasting suffices. Fasting punishes you, but it will not restore your brother! Your privations will be fruitful if you provide for the needs of another. Certainly you have deprived your body, but to whom did you give that which you deprived yourself? How many poor people could be nourished by the meal which you did not take today? Fast, then, in such a way that when another has eaten in your place you may rejoice in the meal you have taken. Then your offering will be received by God.

For the early Christians, "going without meat" was "enabling your neighbor to eat." About the year 128 Aristides, a journalist, explained to Emperor Hadrian the manner in which the Christians lived: "When someone is poor among them who has need of help, they fast for two or three days, and they have the custom of sending him the food which they had prepared for themselves."

In 1950, Pope Pius XII told Christians throughout the world: "What he has rescued from vanity, the faithful Christian will give to charity and thus mercifully provide for . . . the poor. This was the practice in the primitive church. By fasting and abstaining from things that were perfectly permissible, they supplied the sources of charity."

In 1974, eight years after the church removed the Lenten fast, the U.S. Roman Catholic bishops responded to the world food crisis by asking Catholics to fast at least two days a week. The money saved could be contributed to some food-relief organization.

One of the positive developments of the past twenty years is that we have recovered our sense of the ministry of service that is proper to each Christian in virtue of his baptism. Underneath all these statements from our Christian history lies the faith-conviction that fasting *is* ministry, *is* service to others. It is also preparation for ministry because it is discipline in the area of self-denial. Involvement with the needs of others—what ministry is all about—costs us many conveniences and preferences. Making room for the needs of others means denying some of my own needs. And fasting, inasmuch as it represents a reordering of some of our priorities, is ministry when the needs of others are taken into account in our "new agenda."

Ministry requires flexibility to adjust to the needs of others in any given situation. The willingness to go without food when the situation calls for it is one of the faces flexibility in ministry wears.

Ministry requires self-forgetfulness. Fasting as an act of the heart means becoming preöccupied with the Lord himself and then with concerns of his people.

Ministry requires sacrifice. Giving something that matters to us (in this case, food), giving up our own desires in order to help another, is the meaning of sacrifice. "We prove we are God's servants by great fortitude in times of suffering, in time of hardship and distress . . . in laboring, sleepless nights, and in fasting?" (2 Corinthians 6: 4, 5).

All Christians are called to a ministry, to be servants of God. And all ministry is giving. Without almsgiving (in its expanded sense) prayer and fasting tend toward self-centeredness. God has "wired" us in such a way that we grow in love with him in proportion to our love for others. As a poster I saw once put it: "To know God better, love people more." The Apostle John stressed the interrelatedness of love for God and for others this way:

Anyone who says, "I love God," and hates his brother, is a liar, since a man who does not love the brother that he can see cannot love God, whom he has never seen. So this is the commandment that he has given us: that anyone who loves God must also love his brother (1 John 4:20,21).

Fasting, as we have said, is focus upon God. Care for others is not competitive with this, but complementary to it. God has provided a way for us to fast for others, to seek him intently for their needs. In such intercession, the key is identification with them.

Now you together are Christ's body; but each of you is a different part of it. What is more, it is precisely the parts of the body which seem to be the weakest which are the indispensable ones . . . God has arranged the body so that more dignity is given to the parts which are without it, and so that there may not be disagreements inside the body, but that each part may be equally concerned with all the others. If one part is hurt, all parts are hurt with it. If one part is given special honour, all parts enjoy it (1 Corinthians 12:22-27).

Cultural Resistance to Fasting for Others

To reflect upon passages like that, to really take them seriously, is, in our time, to become the rope in a tug-of-war. Pulling us on one end are the new therapies with their refusal to consider moral complexities, the denial of history and a larger community, the disappearance of the Other, the exaggerations of the will, the reduction of all experience to a set of platitudes. And on the other end are moral and historical concerns, conscience, justice, shame, interdependence, and God. With forces like those pulling us in opposing directions, no wonder some of us break, snap, or fray.

What makes fasting for others seem so absurb in the Era of Me is that the new therapies have provided their adherents with a way to avoid the demands of the world, to resist the tug of conscience. They allow us to remain who and what we are, to accept the structured world as it is—but with a new sense of justice and justification, i.e., it all accords with the cosmic law: we are in our proper place; the others are in theirs. In essence, their fate has nothing to do with us. Everyone is responsible for what happens to him or her.

It is the familiar myth of the solitary gunslinger translated into psycho-jargon, the comic-strip story of Captain Marvel made into a slightly more sophisticated legend for adults. This concept of the totally strong, completely self-determined individual who doesn't need anybody is the traditional North American individualistic ethos carried too far—the Clint Eastwood syndrome applied to psychotherapy.

Some of us have probably seen at one time or another this poetic expression of Fritz Perls:

I do my thing, and you do your thing.
I am not in this world to live up to your
expectations,
and you are not in this world to live up
to mine.
You are you and I am I;
If by chance we find each other,
it's beautiful.
If not, it can't be helped.

These lines poignantly express the human needs for independence and self-expression. All of us must have our own thoughts and feelings and must assert our right to express them freely. We must make our own choices and be able to live by them. And no doubt this was the practical good intent Perls had in mind: to expose the clinging dependency and jealous possessiveness which are, in fact, counterfeits of true love. But at the same time his verse opens itself to serious criticism by waving a banner that seems to say: "Do your own thing!"

As Eugene Kennedy writes in his book *Free to Be Human*:

Life cannot be lived as an accidental affair—like a roller derby in which everybody is doing his own thing, with intense absorption, pleasing himself, and to hell with everybody else. And, if by chance, a collision sends a couple into each other's arms for a few moments—that's beautiful?

* * *

When I do my things and you do yours, exactly *where* are we doing these things? In a vacuum so distant that we never meet, or never cross each other's path or need anybody's help? The fact is that part of doing our "thing" is learning to do it with respect for others and their rights.

* * *

And what's wrong with living up to expectations? It is important for parents, teachers, clergymen and spouses to have expectations regarding the behavior of others and not apologize for it. We cripple people and and destroy all possibilities of excellence when we refuse to set standards.

* * *

Excessive subjectivism ignores one of the deepest truths of human existence: to be is to-be-with-others. Perls' credo reflects the human need for independence, but ignores the need for true and deep relationships. Psychologist Walter Tubbs wrote a supplement which redresses the imbalance in the thought of Perls:

If I just do my thing and you do yours,
We stand in danger of losing each other
And ourselves.

I am not in this world to live up to your
expectations;
But I am in this world to confirm you

As a unique human being.
And to be confirmed by you.
We are fully ourselves only in relation
to each other.
The I detached from a Thou
Disintegrates.

I do not find you by chance;
I find you by an active life
Of reaching out.

Rather than passively letting things
happen to me,
I can act intentionally to make them
happen.

I must begin with myself, true;
But I must not end with myself:
The truth begins with two.

The Christian tradition of prayer, fasting, and acts of caring are grounded upon an experience of community, a felt sense of collective responsibility for the fate of each separate other. What is threatening to take its place is a moral vacuum in which others are trapped forever in a "private" destiny, doomed to whatever befalls them. In that void the traditional measures of justice or good vanish completely. The self replaces community, relation, neighbor, providence and God. When the web of reciprocity and relationship is broken, lost is the immense ground of human community.

"I am very much afraid," said Dr. Philippe Rushton, professor of psychology at the University of Western Ontario, "that we may be creating a whole society of self-actualized egoists who are only interested in themselves—and to hell with everyone else!" Altruism, he believes, is "in real danger of declining in our society. All the traditional means of socializing children to be concerned about others are breaking down. The family is less effective today as a means of socializing children than it has ever been. One child in six in North America is being raised by a single parent, often a working single parent. And even in intact families, children have less contact with adults than ever before. At the same time, religion, which used to be embedded in a whole framework of community organizations, is in decline." And as for the schools, they "have just opted out, and refuse to socialize people at all." What has filled the gap? The answer is not reassuring: "To a large extent, television, which socializes children to be aggressive and antisocial," says Rushton.

The bookrack can't be counted upon for respite, either. A sampling of the new wave of self-help books that have been streaming out of the major literary foundries gives: *Power! How to Get It, How to Use It; Winning Through Intimidation; Looking Out for #1; Pulling Your Own Strings; Power, Influence and Control Over People; Women and Power; Big You, Little You; The New Assertive Woman; Think and Grow Rich Action Pack;* and *Success! How Every Man and Woman Can Achieve It.*

The common chord in these books is that wile, guile, manipulation and self-centered one-upmanship are now the recommended routes for rapid ascension in the business world.

Robert J. Ringer, author of *Looking Out for #1*, tells the millions who have bought his books "to learn to ignore your altruistic instincts" and not to concern yourself with honesty since everybody defines that word to suit himself or herself. If you can cow or browbeat the guy you're dealing with before he does it to you, you're a winner. The dictum of Michael Korda, author of the first and last books mentioned above, is that morality is irrelevant to success and that your "interests are nobody else's concern, your gain is inevitably someone else's loss, and your failure is somebody else's success." Korda tells his readers straight out that "it's O.K. to be greedy. It's also O.K. to look out for Number One, to be Machiavellian (if you can get away with it), to recognize that honesty is not always the best policy, to be a winner, and it's always O.K. to be rich." Say it loud: I'm selfish and I'm proud!

Growth and self-actualization are not contra-Gospel in themselves. They are certainly a step along the way to living the Gospel. What the Gospel says is "Love your neighbor as *yourself*," which assumes a certain degree of healthy self-love. There has to be a self before there can be self-sacrifice, before one can choose to put oneself on the line for another. Unless there is a good sense of self-worth, putting the other before myself can't be considered as virtuous behavior. But what the new religion seems to miss is that self-actualization is but a step toward the real goal of interdependence, where you can work cooperatively in relationships that involve strong, balanced, healthy selves who are no longer just worrying about themselves but who don't forget themselves either.

As syndicated *Boston Globe* columnist Ellen Goodman writes of the authors of the self-help books, "There is a difference between climbing the ladder of success and macheteing a path to the top. These writers ... give us a way to live with ourselves, perhaps, but not a way to live with each other. They teach us a whole lot more about 'failure' than about success."

For another criterion of success and failure, try the letter of Paul to the Church at Philippi:

> If our life in Christ means anything to you, if love can persuade at all, or the Spirit that we have in common, or any tenderness and sympathy, then be united in your convictions and united in your love, with a common purpose and a common mind. That is the one thing which would make me completely happy. There must be no competition among you, no conceit; but everybody is to be self-effacing. Always consider the other person to be better than yourself, so that nobody thinks of his own interests first but everybody thinks of other people's interests instead. In your minds you must be the same as Christ Jesus:

> > His state was divine,
> > yet he did not cling
> > to his equality with God
> > but emptied himself
> > to assume the condition of a slave,
> > and became as men are,
> > and being as all men are,
> > he was humbler yet,
> > even to accepting death,
> > death on a cross.

> (Philippians 2:3-8)

Fasting at God's Initiative

The primary self to be transcended in fasting is *my*self (me!). Fasting that is pleasing to God and not merely an exercise of vanity or mere preservation of temporal life is accompanied by a spirit of humility, repentance, and true sincerity of heart. Fundamentally, fasting represents offering oneself to God in a spirit of openness and readiness, inviting the action of his Spirit. Such an impulse must first come from God and not be of our own planning. The movement and timing of the Lord are important so that our fasting may be a true, religious act of loving worship and self-surrender. It must be the Holy Spirit who leads us into the deeper Christian values of fasting. This prevents fasting from becoming a technique taken on solely for health purposes or expanded consciousness or for whatever purpose that could so easily become another idol in ourselves. Unless we are responding from the heart to an initiative from God, our fasting will be motivated by self-interest. It may look like a dedicated religious act, but the motive of our hearts will be to please ourselves.

Fasting is not merely renunciation or self-discipline, arduously forged by the human will. Important as virtue is, seeking it too selfconsciously can lead to a very subtle but serious error: thinking of virtue as something that depends on my effort alone. That mode of thinking was tabled as a heresy in 529 at the Council of Orange and called Pelagianism, after a British monk named Pelagius, who thought that the human person is in possession of his full integrity— even after the Fall. We can accomplish our own salvation by ourselves, according to Pelagius. Adam and Eve gave us a bad example, Jesus a good example. Follow Christ's. That's all there is to it. We need no other support than that of our own freedom and courage.

The high-schooler may resolve to add an inch to his biceps before football season begins. A forty-year-old woman may decide to jog or swim three times a week to keep fit. A businessman may set a date to quit drinking. These and similar goals depend largely on our determination to follow through on the goal we have chosen.

But virtue is not simply a matter of will power. According to the Gospels, Jesus did not become angry with many people. But there was one crowd he constantly rebuked: those who were self-righteous, who thought they had it made with God because of their own efforts. In the Gospel of Luke (18:14), the man who self-righteously fasted twice a week and then thanked God that he was not like everyone else was severely criticized by our Lord. Such "virtue" is usually concerned that people notice it, that it be recognized and praised. Genuine virtue is God's grace in action, and not simply the product of one's free will which, by the way, is itself God's gift.

Fasting is an action that flows from experiencing what it means to live in Christ: "All I want is to know Christ and the power of his resurrection and to share his sufferings by reproducing the pattern of his death. That is the way I can hope to take my place in the resurrection of the dead" (Philippians 3:10-13). The Spirit teaches us how to integrate the different dimensions of our life as spiritual flesh. The Spirit teaches us to fast so that such an experience under Her power will engender a state of balance and truthfulness, i.e., humility, which enables us to direct our lives harmoniously toward God and our neighbor. Throughout the Bible God has clearly encouraged us to fast as one of the best means to enter into purity of heart. Ultimately the experience of such purity of heart is found in observing the traditional forms of ascetical practices that God in the Bible and through his church and his saints has exhorted us to perform. Fasting always has been and will always be a vital way of growing into the integrated person we are called to be in the Spirit of Jesus.

Fasting for Others at God's Initiative

When we transcend ourselves in fasting by focusing upon God, we do not stay there. The shift of focus from ourselves and what we are doing, to God enables us to receive a further shift in focus: upon the needs of others. Once God has our attention, he can shape and affect our perception of the needs of others. It has been the constant experience of men and women who fast that abstaining from food not only frees them to focus upon God with fresh intensity, but opens avenues of spiritual perception and understanding that are not available during the rush of routine living. They find a clarity of direction and quickening of spirit as they focus upon God by deliberate discipline.

Fasting itself is not the power—God is. When our hearts are freed from debris and clutter, the Holy Spirit can once again flow through us freely. We become a clearer witness to God's presence and action in the world. Our usefulness as his channels is increased.

Because fasting increases our awareness of God's initiative, it consequently intensifies the confidence with which we go forward into prayer and ministry. As we set aside the many other stimuli that beckon for our attention, it is easier for us to distinguish the direction of the Lord. The problem is never with God's speaking, but with our hearing. We have to turn aside from the clamor and really listen. Our sense of confidence in the Spirit who leads us is usually diminished because we dissipate our energies and attention in so many activities and directions that we lose our focus. Loss of focus is reflected as unsureness, indecisiveness, lack of confidence. We second-guess our

118

instincts and the inner suggestions of spirit, and soon find ourselves bewildered by seeming ineffectiveness in ministries to which God had seemed to lead us to clearly at an earlier time. Since fasting essentially relates to a focus of the heart and spirit, it is important not only as a preparation for ministry (preparing us for sacrificial giving through a discipline of self-denial), and not only as ministry itself, but it also helps after the fashion of a compass to keep us from getting lost on the road to which we have been directed.

But the compass itself has a compass. The gauge God has provided for fasting is its results in our own lives and its effectiveness in relation to others around us. If fasting is doing its work of liberating our focus from self-preoccupation, this will manifest itself in mercy and compassion toward those around us. We will be moved from within to give what we are receiving from God.

Fasting which is a response to God's initiative will result in practical outreach. We will respond to the need we see, not just to God in prayer (though that is certainly important). Our lives will be marked by concrete caring responses for others. Fasting must deal with reality. it does not skirt issues. It is not an interior escape. The fast God has chosen prepares us within in such a way that we can be used to bring about change in outward circumstances. Inner liberation spills over into outward acts of caring. Fasting is directly related to social responsibility.

> This is the fast that pleases me
> —It is the Lord Yahweh who speaks—
> to break unjust fetters
> and undo the thongs of the yoke,
> to let the oppressed go free,
> and break every yoke,
> to share your bread with the hungry,
> and shelter the homeless poor,
> to clothe the man you see to be naked
> and to turn not from your own kin (Isaiah 59:6-8).

Isaiah's verbs all go outward in the action of sharing. As we noted earlier, identification with the needy is the key. The kind of sharing Isaiah speaks of cannot be done without deep personal investment in the concerns of the other. This is the kind of caring wherein the needs of the other become my own. The key which unlocks the chest of my own resources is compassion.

119

In Isaiah's phrase, "do not turn from your own flesh," there is contained a whole theology, an entire mind-set, a complete system of values, a vision of life. The Hebrew word for "flesh" in this passage includes a broad scope of meaning that encompasses my body-spirit, my self, my relatives, and all my kin—that is to say: humanity. "Do not turn from your own flesh."

Reaffirming our Connectedness

We are perhaps at this moment in our reflection at the farthest possible point from the rampant philosophy of our era. In the Era of Me, there is a tyrannical refusal to acknowledge the existence of a world larger than the self, the denial (by implication) of the necessity of human community or relationship.

Peter Marin in an article entitled "The New Narcissism" tells of a conversation he had with a man much taken with mysticism and "spirituality" who was telling him about his sense of another reality:

"I know there is something outside of me," he said. "I can feel it. I know it is there. But what is it?"

"It may not be a mystery," I said. "Perhaps it is the world."

That startled him. He had meant something more magical than that, more exotic and grand, something "above" rather than all around him. It had never occurred to him that what might be calling to him from beyond the self were the worlds of community and value, the worlds of history and action—all of them waiting to be entered not as a saint or a mystic, but in a way more difficult still: as a moral man or woman among other persons, with a person's real and complex nature and needs. Those worlds had been closed to him, had receded from consciousness as he had ceased to inhabit them fully or responsibly or lovingly, and so he felt their ghostly presence as something distant and mysterious, as a dream in which he had no actual existence.

Marin goes on to remark that it is as if each of us had at the same time a smaller and larger self, as if we inhabited at the same moment a smaller and larger world. The smaller world, of course, is the one familiar to us, the world of the individual ego and our friendships, a reality acknowledged by our habits of thought and by our institutions and therapies. But we also inhabit a larger and *unrealized* world, one in which every gesture becomes significant precisely because it is understood to bind us to the lives of invisible others.

We have forgotten—or were never aware—that almost without exception the visionary experiences of Indian cultures are a collective work, prepared, defined and sustained by the community, by a world view which is, in effect, the product of cooperative labor. When they came back from their vision quests, the American Indians recited their newly made poems or sang their songs to the tribe, feeding back to it the shared truths of a solitude that was *not* separate, but shared.

We forget that love, that sense of lived relation, is at the heart not only of tribal lore, but at the center of the legends of most cultures. Odysseus surrounded by comrades seeking to return to his home; Gilgmesh driven to seek the secret of immortality by the death of Enkidu, his friend. Both of them are moved by what lies behind all myth and long-lived culture: the felt sense of relation and reciprocity.

We have, in Marin's words, "an appetence for Good: the needful reaching out for a life in a larger world. We are moved toward that world by the inner force Freud called Eros: the desire for relation is as as much at work in our need for community and moral significance as it is in our need for coupled love." Seen in this way, human fulfillment hinges on much more than our usual notions of private pleasure or self-actualization, for both of those in their richest forms are not possible without communion and community. To be deprived of these latter is "to be deprived of a part of the self," Marin reflects, "and to turn away from them is to betray not only the world but also the self, for it is only in the realms in which others exist that one can come to understand the ways in which the nature of each individual existence is in many ways a collective act, the result of countless other lives. . . .Every privilege, every object, every 'good' comes to us as the result of a human harvest, the shared labor of others: the language we use and the beliefs we hold and the ways we experience ourselves. Each of these involves a world of others into which we are entered every moment of our lives."

Surely we have always known this: that each individual existence is in many ways a collective act, the result of countless other lives. It is a truth that needs only a moment's reflection to bear it out: the husband and wife who sacrifice their own ambitions and their material assets in order to provide a better future for their children ... the soldier who risks his life, or perhaps consciously sacrifices it, in battle . . . the man who devotes his life to some struggle for "his people" that cannot possibly be won in his lifetime . . . people who buy life insurance or leave wills . . . most women, upon becoming pregnant for the first time . . . are people who conceive of themselves, however subconsciously, as part of a connected lifestream. Just as something of their ancestors lives on in them, so will something of them live on in their children, on in their people, their race, their community. They live as if they are living their ancestors' lives and their offsprings' lives and perhaps their neighbors' lives as well.

In an article in *Psychology Today* entitled "Why Some People Can't Love," Linda Wolfe interviews Dr. Otto Kernberg, a leading authority and theorist on narcissism. He makes a point that human nature seeks its own fulfillment, in spite of the experiment that society may be engaged in at any given time (e.g., the "human potential movement"):

Wolfe: It sounds to me as if you are saying that while society may change, neither human nature nor the concept of what is most likely to satisfy human longings changes—no matter what society decrees. You are suggesting that it is a given fact that in order to feel fulfilled as human beings, we must feel deeply for others, whether our society promotes attachment or urges us away from it.

Kernberg: Yes, I think so. All other things being equal, there is something that happens to one in a deep relationship with someone else which brings great satisfaction to the individual. It has been called transcendence, the sense of extending beyond oneself and feeling a sense of unity with all others who have lived and loved and suffered before—whether it is one's parents or people throughout history. And when that can't be attained, one feels emptiness and chronic dissatisfaction.

Wolfe: Then you think there's no real danger of narcissism becoming the prevailing trait of our society because the individual psyche will rebel against it?

Kernberg: Yes. Individuals will simply continue to choose the pattern that fulfills them, despite what society promulgates.

Fasting In Unity

Christians have continued to choose the "patterns" of prayer, fasting, and caring behavior in their quest for fulfillment. Through the ages of Christian experience, it has come to be accepted that fasting, to be truly Christian, must be characterized by a radical turning of ourselves to God with a corresponding openness to love and serve our neighbor. If these two elements are lacking, fasting may have some beneficial effects physiologically, but it will not be a true religious act.

When, through fasting, we let go of some of that independent control we have so long exerted over our lives, we move on to a different level of consciousness. One of its fruits is a deeper sense of oneness with every human being. In the experience of creaturely poverty that fasting brings, there is a sense of gentleness and kinship with every God-created being that exists. It is the kind of experience that Adrian Van Kaam speaks of in his book *On Being Yourself*:

> I find in my deepest self the mystery of my own Origin, which is the Origin of all that is. In these depths I feel at-one with God. I feel also at-one with every person and thing that emerges from the same Divine Ground. On the deepest level of my life, it is no longer possible to distinguish a vertical relationship to God and a horizontal relationship to man. I cannot see one without at least implicitly experiencing the other.

When I realize who God is and who I myself am; when I realize the utter gratuity of all creation, a total thanksgiving wells up from the very depths of a grateful, receiving being. All is gift, and gratefully received. Greed is gone. Nothing is taken for granted. All is reverenced. There is a loving care for every person and everything. Sufficiency is more than enough, for it is more than is deserved. It is what is wanted for all. And what one has is shared with all, with that end in view. It is staggering to realize that God has so disposed that the unfolding of his sharing of his own goodness should be shaped in some way by our good will or lack of it. But such is the way God seems to have ordered things. And hence with compassion and sensitivity the Christian must constantly be involved in justice-serving behavior.

This new-found consciousness renders us particularly sensitive to the physical, psychic, and spiritual needs of our fellow human beings. It becomes, for example, more and more difficult to eat and drink excessively (or even moderately, of costly, delicate foods and drinks), knowing that others are starving. There is a desire to want to share what God has given. Lanza del Vasto, one of Gandhi's

123

disciples, once wrote: "When you think of men starving in the world you are forced to cry out for them with a more sensitive heart. One who fasts is made transparent. Others appear to him transparent. Their sufferings enter into him and he is without defense against them."

As a friend once wrote to me:

> Fasting is a way of identifying with all the suffering peoples of the world, especially those dying of hunger. We tend to forget the pain of the world if we are always very comfortable. My fasting helps to remind me of the Christ who is suffering in many people all around the world.

Through the centuries the fast has been used as a means of drawing communities of people together, providing them with a common experience and the opportunity to share that experience. Lent. The Day of Atonement. Ramadan.

Fasting has also been used to organize groups around socialchange movements. Many leaders of such groups have fasted as an act of exemplary sacrifice and discipline, often dramatizing an issue and bringing public attention to bear upon it. Mahatma Gandhi was a major practitioner of this approach through his fasts for Indian independence.

Gandhi's example has been a profound inspiration to other leaders of social reform in places as disparate as Sicily and California. In Sicily, Danilo Dolci rallied peasants around his fasts, inspiring them to throw off the yoke of oppression; in California, Cesar Chavez through his fasting example coalesced the efforts of migrants to form a farm-worker's union.

The last decade has seen many people take up fasting as an expression of moral indignation and protest. The dramatic "hunger strike" of fasting in public to protest political or social injustice has claimed many participants during the civil-rights movement, the Vietnam War, and the protest against nuclear-energy power plants. People fasted to express outrage at the nation's spiraling defense budget. Members of Christian communities fasted to signal their chagrin with the opulent living quarters of church leaders and church spending policies. It draws attention to a cause and often results in remedial action. At the present time one of the leading exponents of fasting for this purpose has been entertainer Dick Gregory. In fact, regular fasting has so changed his own attitudes about eating and

124

health that he has become an active advocate of new approaches to dieting and nutrition.

Some would see the remedial action merely in political terms, i.e., a fast carried on too long will cross the line into starvation, and those at whom the fast is directed do not want to jeopardize their position further by creating martyrs. Others would see the fast as a moral force, an effective instrument of spiritual intercession which cries out to God with earnestness to change the hearts of those at whom the fast is directed. And still others would see fasting as certainly possessing but going beyond mere moral force to become an instrument of practical, concrete action. An outstanding example of this latter vision is found in an organization called Bread for the World.

Bread for the World

A Christian organization dedicated to fighting world hunger, "Bread for the World" has as part of its campaign to persuade every North American Christian to abstain from meat three days a week as a way of aiding nations of the Third World. The rationale behind this is that each U.S. citizen consumes on the average about 1,850 pounds of grain per year, compared to 400 pounds in poor countries, mainly because we consume most of ours *indirectly* as meat and dairy products. According to the U.S. Department of Agriculture, the average pound of edible beef in the U.S. represents seven pounds of grain. Hence, cutting back on grain-fed meat makes sense. President Ford asked Americans to cut down on food consumption by 5 percent. That amount seems negligible and hard to measure. But, put in different terms, if we fast one day a week, we are reducing our food consumption by almost 15 percent! Over a year's time this would add up to almost two months of foodless days. However, abstaining from meat three days a week or two months of foodless days each year does not automatically transfer food to hungry people.

This is where the plot thickens. This is where the calling of the followers of Jesus, who claim a global citizenship ("God so loved the *world*") takes on an added responsibility. "Feed the hungry," Jesus said.

"But how?" we ask. We see' the development of new farming technologies, the rapid growth of transportation and communication. We know that food *can* be grown and *can* be distributed. What stops it from happening?

To answer this question, representatives of 130 national governments assembled for the first time in Rome in 1974 under UN auspices for the World Food Conference. The Conference proposed a world food-reserve program coordinated internationally, but with supplies held nationally. In order to coordinate this and other related proposals, the United Nations established the World Food Council, with headquarters in Rome. The Conference gave us an important insight into the complexity and political nature of food distibution. It called for broader social and economic reforms that will have to occur within poor countries if hunger is to be noticeably reduced, including land and tax reforms that would benefit small farm-holders and landless peasants. It asked for a new economic relationship between rich and poor countries in order to stem the widening economic gap that separates them. This points toward areas such as trade, investment and the monetary system. Actions at this level are often the most important and difficult of all.

Seeing an exposition of the problem of hunger in the world on such a scale makes us realize that we will not deal effectively with hunger simply through private acts of charity. It may be possible for us, for example, to feed a hungry family or two near us (something which is well worth doing), without altering at all the conditions that brought about their hunger. If we really care about hungry people, we must eventually ask *why* they are hungry.

They are hungry because they are poor. Which means we cannot come to terms with hunger unless we deal with poverty. We are then confronted with some of the harsh realities that explain why some have and others have not. In the end, in order to make lasting gains against hunger, the concern from which charity flows must also give rise to justice.

The same amount of food that is feeding 210 million Americans would feed 1.5 billion Chinese on an average Chinese diet, according to Dr. Jean Mayler. In other words, it is conceivable that we could get along in good health (the Chinese diet is considered to be one of the healthiest in the world) on one-seventh of the food we are now consuming.

The fact that 5 percent of the human race consumes more marketable wealth than does the poor 70 percent of the world has prompted many to re-examine their style of living and shift toward a more sparing, less materialistic way of life. The Christian tradition has valued (though Christians have not always practiced) simplicity of life and voluntary poverty, a gospel ideal drawn from Jesus himself who had "nowhere to lay his head." It is a life-style expressed daily in the lives of millions of ordinary Christians who have chosen to share what they have with others in response to the Gospel. The transfer of resources involved is relatively limited. The chief value in this lifestyle is spiritual and symbolic—which is not to say it isn't real or valuable. It simply is to recognize that the power behind such commitment consists in lives that are placed more fully at the disposal of God and other people, and in keeping alive for others a sense of proportion.

The point to be made here is that going without food for a day a week, and contributing to a good cause the money that you would otherwise have spent on your meals, fails to go to the heart of the problem. It is like swinging at the ball but only nicking a piece of it, as opposed to hitting it squarely. To "hit it squarely," we need to move from the personal to the public realm on this problem. If that move does not happen, the grain that I save by giving up meat three times a week may be sold to feed *livestock* in a faraway country, or simply not be planted next year by farmers who are worried about low prices. Food will reach hungry people only if government policies see to its proper production and distribution. An adjustment in eating habits without responsible citizenship may prescribe failure and hurt farmers.

To the question, "What can I do besides give?" the World Food Conference implicitly told the average citizen: influence government policy. That answer should not discourage giving on the personal, neighborhood, city level; but it tells us that it is necessary to move beyond the adjusted-life-style approach if we are really interested in doing something about feeding the hungry. Adopting a more modest life-style can be a powerful witness in the struggle against hunger, if efforts to change public policy accompany it. But we can't afford to stop at the level of life-style. While life-style changes appeal as immediate, personal responses, they can also lull us into a false sense of fulfillment. Cutting down on our food intake, or giving up certain types of food because most of the world's poor cannot afford to eat in the manner of North Americans, may be morally satisfying, but unless it is accompanied by more positive steps, it may do nothing more on the practical level of feeding the hungry than put people out of work.

If, however, I use my lunch hour on a fast day to write a letter that tells my representative in Congress or Parliament what I think of our public policy regarding food distribution and what I want our country to do—that is the kind of response to world hunger that brings together life-style adjustment (my fast) with positive action (my letters—written on time freed-up by my fast) to influence government policy. Our sense of responsibility must become sufficiently deep to encompass both.

The same principle (We Can Deal With Both) applies to the charity-begins-at-home argument that says "Shouldn't we eliminate hunger here before we try to solve the problem worldwide?" There's no need to put domestic hunger against world hunger in an either/or playoff. We can deal with both.

"The urgent need," says Arthur Simon, Executive Director of Bread for the World and author of the book by the same name, "is not for churches *as churches* to enter the political fray (although they must take moral stands), but for Christians *as citizens* to exercise their renewed consciences and contact decision-makers." Simon recommends that people become a voice for the hungry to their member of government.

A single action by Parliament or Congress, one decision by the President or Prime Minister can multiply—or undo—many times over the effect of all our voluntary contributions derived from fast days. To make an offering in church for world relief is good, but it doesn't go far enough if we leave the big decisions up to political representatives without letting them know what we want. Our citizenship is our most powerful tool against hunger. Not to exercise it is taken as indifference when policies are being worked out; it leaves leaders free to make decisions by other standards and hungry people become victims of political lobbying.

"Each of us helps to decide how our nation should use its power and wealth in a hungry world," Simon writes. "If we choose not to get involved, we are making the kind of decisions that lock people into hunger. Put another way, saying nothing to political leaders *is* saying something to them. We usually get the kind of leadership we ask for on this, and if we ask for none, that is what we can expect . . . We do not have to let the trends tell us what to do. Despair is unbelief. Ordinary people *can* help the nation reach out to a hungry world. To do so we will have to add to our contributions for world relief the offering of our citizenship."

Thus, in a very real way, the nature of our shared human world does depend on our actions and words. We can destroy it and kin of our own flesh not only with bombs, but through our failure to inhabit it as justly and responsibly as we should.

The Gospel and Human Justice

This is what the Lord asks of you, only this:
to act justly,
to love tenderly,
and to walk humbly with your God (Micah 6:8).

Our churches are not going to *impose* fasting and abstinence upon us today. But true Christian concern will urge us to fast and to use our time and energy to touch the hearts of civil leaders so that they become vitally concerned with the realities of poverty and starvation that involve so many millions of our brothers and sisters in the human family.

Our experience of God's love, heightened by the clarity of perception that comes from regular fasting, sets us free to care about others. When their need confronts us, we want to know what we can do to help. And if that concern is genuine, we will want the action we take to do more than make us feel good or bring only temporary relief to the people in need. We will want our action to deal with their need as effectively as possible. Dealing effectively with hunger pushes us into the public-policy arena, into questions of social justice.

Our guidelines in that arena are drawn from the values of Sacred Scripture, the value that God places on human life and the belief that "the earth is the Lord's and the fullness thereof." We affirm the right to food of every man, woman, and child on earth. We want to overcome a situation that flagrantly violates the humanity of the hungry. We want to see those sons and daughters of the same heavenly Father as our own enjoy their full human dignity as his children.

As believers we do not root our hope in the latest projections of the United Nations or some social scientist's analysis of how things may turn out in fifteen or fifty years. We root our hope in God and believe that the future is with his reign on this earth. We believe that no efforts consistent with this hope are wasted. Our efforts are signs of the presence of God's Spirit and through them God does his work. The Christian understanding of human nature—flawed, but capable of good under grace—should spare us from the disillusionments that make so many of today's crusaders tomorrow's cynics. And our

Christian hope should give us staying power long after many others have become disgruntled and gone on to another cause. We need to remember that to break bread at the Lord's table and to say "Amen" to the Bread of Life is to take responsibility for his Body in all its members and to make a commitment to enable hungry brothers and sisters to break bread, too.

6 Holiness Is Wholeness: Fasting Is Fitness

> *Let me put it like this: if you are guided by the Spirit*
> *you will be in no danger of yielding to self-indulgence,*
> *since self-indulgence is the opposite of the Spirit; the*
> *Spirit is totally against such a thing, and it is precisely*
> *because the two are so opposed that you do not always*
> *carry out your good intentions. . . . When self-indul-*
> *gence is at work, the results are obvious: fornication,*
> *gross indecency, and sexual irresponsibility; disagree-*
> *ments, factions, envy, drunkenness, orgies and similar*
> *things. . . . What the Spirit brings is very different:*
> *love, joy, peace, patience, kindness, goodness, truth-*
> *fulness, gentleness, and self-control. . . . Since the*
> *Spirit is our life, let us be directed by the Spirit*
> (Galatians 5:16-26).

Spirituality and Our Bodies

Spirituality is simply the art of growing closer to God. For the Christian that means following Christ's footsteps to the Father in the power of the Spirit.

A wholesome spirituality *begins* with being comfortable with our bodies. Unless I am comfortable with my own body and love it, striving for wholeness or union with God (which is what spirituality is all about) easily becomes an escape from the body, an unnatural splitting of body and spirit.

Growth in spirituality is the slow work of God's grace helping us to fully accept and harmoniously integrate all the dimensions of our selves. When bodiliness and spiritedness become in my consciousness but two dimensions of my one being, I am on the way to holiness, which is wholeness. These two dimensions of myself must merge in my consciousness and become one, just as they are in reality. I am not body *and* soul (two things), I am spirited flesh (or an

131

enfleshed spirit): one reality. When I embrace that incredibly rich and exciting reality and love it, I am accepting and appreciating the self God has given me in all its totality.

When I was doing my graduate studies in theology, a professor surprised our sacraments class one day by giving us the homework assignment of standing stark naked in front of a full-length mirror and just looking at ourselves from every angle for fifteen minutes.

There were actually several methods to his madness. Firstly, he wanted us to confront within ourselves in dramatic fashion our own conviction about the goodness of material creation. The concrete world around us is the stuff of the sacraments: bread, wine, water, oil. If creation is not good, how can the sacraments be good? We were eventually to study in the history of the sacraments how the times when sacraments took a lesser place in the life of the church were precisely those times when there was a lack of appreciation for the goodness of creation. When material creation was not seen to mediate God's presence, there arose the problem of dualism: spirit is good, matter is evil. Or, put differently, "if I can only become spiritual, then that dirty old body will somehow go away!" During these periods of human history, marriage was little more than a necessary institution for the propagation of the race, and sex was sinful if you enjoyed it too much.

Secondly, our professor wanted us to come to grips with the psychological reality that the attitude we have toward our physical appearance often masks attitudes deeper within us that concern our very selves. Our attitudes about our *selves* are "coded" into the image we have of our bodies and can be found there. The years of positive and/or negative messages we have absorbed affect the way we see ourselves through our outward image, the body. And seeing the body as an outer image of an inner self is already a division. I *am* my body, and therefore I must embrace my body if I am going to embrace myself.

And thirdly, as long as we proclaim the resurrection of the body from the dead and life everlasting in a glorified embodied spirit, we had better be deeply convinced of the importance and place of caring for our bodies. It would be somewhere between humorous and tragic if the Word of God becomes human, redeems us in and through his bodiliness, rises from the tomb and appears in a glorified bodily state only to see some of his followers striving to become "spiritual" or "Christlike" by rejecting the bodily dimension of their lives and selves!

So that night, in many different houses around the city, a young man or a young woman was standing in front of a full-length mirror trying to hear God say, "I love what you see." Only then could we look again and be able to say to ourselves, "I love what I see."

If we live with this sense of our own goodness and worth, each of us can say with the American poet Emily Dickinson, "Instead of getting to heaven at last / I'm going all along!" In that final line of one of her poems, she gives us a terse, modern and wholesome summary of the spiritual life. Heaven is not a time or a place where I will finally escape the tension of living in "this body." Eternity is already begun. Each one of us is a work of art, an original by God. My personal history of salvation is the story of my struggle to accept that, believe in it, and respond to it with my whole soul and my whole mind and my whole body. Which is to say, as a whole person. Soul, mind, and body are a mini-trinity: a unity, one person. Living from this perspective results in unifying my life. There is no split between my day-to-day living and my spiritual life; what is good for me physically is good for my self, and what is good for me spiritually is good for my self. When everything is swept up into the spiritual life like this, I'm not just "getting to heaven at last, I'm going all along." The going itself is the path, and the journey is joyful.

Murray Bodo, a long-time spiritual director for hundreds of men and women, provides some guidelines for a modern spirituality in an article entitled "Advice for Spiritual Joggers." In speaking of the books written on spirituality in the last fifteen years, he notes that none of them changes the essentials of spiritual conversion, such as repentance, detachment, prayer, penance, overcoming selfishness, and living in charity, but that there is a different emphasis. He illustrates with penance:

> Penance does not consist of punishing myself, or making prayer a time of self-analysis, or seeing the body as *the* great enemy in overcoming selfishness. Penance now is turning from self to God, letting him work in my life, believing that he loves me and has saved me and is saving me each day. And the business of modern spirituality is to get into contact with what God is doing in my life by lovingly embracing myself and others. Embracing is emphasized instead of renouncing, although renunciation is always involved in the selfless embrace.

Holiness is Whole-ly Loving

When asked, "Master, what is the greatest commandment of the Law?" Jesus responded, "You shall love the Lord your God with all your heart, all your soul, and all your strength. And the second resembles it: you must love your neighbor as yourself" (Matthew 22:34-40).

It is only when I am one, not divided, with myself that I can love my neighbor properly. If my self is divided, so will be my love for another. If I love my spirit, and hate my body, then when I love and embrace you, you will not feel loved at all; I am loving a disembodied spirit inside of you that is God-like in spite of your "bad" body.

But there is no such thing. If I truly love you, then I love *you*, whole and entire, just as you are. If I am to love you that way, I have first to love myself that way. "Love your neighbor *as* yourself." That means that I do not live for the promise of some tomorrow or the potential that some day may be revealed in me. It means that I usually feel about myself, as I am, with the same warm and glad emotions that we feel when we meet someone whom we really like and admire. Loving myself means that I am sensitively aware of all that is good in me, from the little things like the way I smile or walk, through the natural talents I have been given, to the virtues I have worked to cultivate.

God's grace does not simply cover a sorry mess, and human nature is not totally corrupt. People holding this pessimistic view tend to recoil from their own drives and impulses as dangerous and evil. The good news of Jesus and the message of his incarnation is that we are basically good, though wounded by sin, and that we can be healed by his amazing grace. He has destroyed sin and death, and he is healing the division within us. Jesus encourages us to have a wholesome love and respect for ourselves.

Fasting as an Exercise of Love, Respect, and Care for Ourselves

A friend of mine was given the gift of a new ten-speed bicycle. He kept it in his garage. I mentioned to him once that he should get a lock for it because a lot of people come and go in the downtown area where he lives and the garage door doesn't represent much security. For whatever reason, he never did get a lock, and he eventually lost his bike. It was stolen from the garage.

I'm not sure whether he was ever really very interested in biking, and it may well be that, although it was a lovely gift, it may not have been something that he valued having all that much. Whereas he's a dedicated jogger, he used his bike only a few times. That may have something to do with why he never got a lock as further insurance against losing it.

For me there's a parallel in the way we care for our mental and physical health. God gives us a gift of a marvelous and delicate embodied spirit. It's brand new, with everything functioning perfectly. And he says, "O.K., it's yours now. You take care of it. You love it and respect it and care for it. If you don't, you'll lose it."

One of the ways by which we can exercise care and respect and love for ourselves is fasting.

Normally, the body is constantly working to digest foods, eliminate wastes, fight diseases, replenish worn-out cells, and nourish the blood. Of these, masticating and digesting the food is its biggest chore. When there is no food to digest, our energy is turned with fuller force upon the other "projects." Giving our bodies a chance to eliminate the toxic wastes that have been stored in the tissues or held in the pockets of the intestines and which interfere with the proper digestive and blood-building functions is an act of care for ourselves.

Dr. Alexis Carrel, the geneticist and Nobel Prize winner, describes what happens in fasting in his book *Man, the Unknown*:

> The sugar of the liver and the fat of the subcutaneous deposit are mobilized, and also the proteins of the muscles and the glands. All the organs sacrifice their own substances in order to maintain blood, heart, and brain in a normal condition. Fasting purifies and profoundly modifies our tissues.

To test the efficacy of fasting, one has only to abstain from food, with the exception of water, for a day or two; note how the tongue (being an organ of elimination) becomes thickly coated with mucous, and how the odor of decaying materials is on the breath. The body is simply taking advantage of an opportunity to eliminate an excess of stored-up wastes that were clogging up the tissues and bloodstream, affecting the functioning of the lungs, kidneys, bladder, stomach, intestinal tract and just about every organ of the body. Following each fast with a cleansing diet of fruits and greenleaf vegetables, eaten either in their natural or cooked state, is a healing and health-restoring act of stewardship over the gift we have been given.

Why Deliberate Cleansing Measures Are More Important Today

Scientists estimate that an inhabitant of the industrial city stands a better than average chance of contracting a deadly lung disease or suffering from heart trouble, just by breathing polluted air. There is hardly a large city where the exhaust emissions from the automobiles alone hasn't become dangerous to the well-being of the people who live there. When one adds to that the soot and smoke from the chimneys of our industrial era, the by-products of industry released into the air, one begins to realize that there is simply more of a need today consciously and deliberately to give ourselves a chance to purify our bodies from these poisons. Our water is so filthy that powerful chemicals are used to make it fit to drink. This year's crop of fruit and vegetables are exposed to more poisonous pesticides than ever before. There are more than a thousand synthetic food additives dumped onto our food supply (take, for example, your basic loaf of commercially refined white bread: it has been treated, bleached, colored, enriched, purified, softened, preserved, flavored, and given a fresh odor—all by synthetic chemicals).

A twenty-four to thirty-six hour weekly fast will help you get rid of as much commercial dirt as possible. It's a life-supporting act.

Sickness is nature's way of indicating that we are filled with toxic wastes and internal poison. When they collect there in various parts of ourselves, we feel uncomfortable pressures and we suffer from aches and pains. In fasting, we are working with nature to help expel the accumulated encumbrances.

Some Areas of Particular Health Concern

As Otto H. F. Buchinger, M.D., noted, in his book *Everything You Want to Know About Fasting*, next to the influences of living in a nervous, anxious, cramped or anger-ridden atmosphere, overfeeding and wrong-feeding, too little exercise as well as tobacco and alcohol contribute decisively to all kinds of diseases and sufferings. The organism's many possibilities of helping itself without an illness becoming manifest and of putting itself in order again are sooner or later exhausted. The body's processes of combustion and energy transformation degenerate. Changes occur in the capillaries and there are general or local disturbances in circulation. The harmonious working together of all the organs, parts, tissues, and glands is upset.

We are taken unawares by a surprise packet of ills. Toxic substances have found their way into the body. Fatigue, headaches, excesses of uric acid and rheumatic poisons, abdominal distention, feelings of anxiety and oppression of the heart and lungs announce themselves. The poisons of metabolism are deposited in numerous tissues, organs and joints, spreading infections. A human wreck, pain-ridden, suffering, tired of life, is the result.

Overweight. We have absorbed the at-large view that the body must have a fattening oversupply of nourishment to strengthen its defenses and build up its powers of resistance. However, the "save-for-a-rainy-day" approach doesn't apply in health care. We have learned from actuarial tables compiled by major insurance companies around the world that desirable weight for an adult is considerably less than average weight. The difference is about ten pounds. The insurance companies invested in the study because they had already noted that one tends to live longer if one is thinner. It has been estimated that some 65-70 percent of the men, women, and children in the United States are overweight. More than half of those could be officially classified as obese.

Overweight is a hazard to health and life. It's like not locking your bicycle: There's a good chance you'll lose it. For every cubic inch of fat on the overweight person, the body has to develop 700 miles of fine tubes to nourish and sustain the excess fat. Obviously, this puts a tremendous strain on the breathing apparatus and normal function of the heart. Pulse and blood pressure rise to dangerous heights, which threaten serious internal damage to ourselves. Even death. "Man digs his grave with his knife and fork," according to an old saying.

One of the things that the nutritional experts Arnold Ehret and Paul Bragg both emphasize very strongly is that we should never force ourselves to eat unless we are truly hungry and a keen relish for food exists. Otherwise, we may add work to an already-overworked digestive tract, pushing it to the point of exhaustion and collapse. We oftentimes think that increasing the quantity of food will give us more energy, when what actually happens is that we end up feeling very enervated and listless. Overeating paralyzes us, and then we experience the need for something to "get us going," so we reach for the stimulants: coffee, tea, tobacco, and alcohol.

Most of us have regular eating routines of breakfast, lunch, and dinner every day, and we eat regardless of whether we are all that hungry or not. Most of us probably don't even look at it in terms of whether we're hungry, and off we go on the lunch hour or to the supper table.

Bragg believes that it would be healthier for us to skip breakfast. With full awareness of the many nutritional books which say that breakfast is "the most important meal of the day," I present Bragg's interesting hypothesis for the reader's own consideration.

In Bragg's estimation, we've been brainwashed to think that we must have meals by the clock. Through reflex conditioning, the stomach expects food before going to work in the morning. But as far as his knowledge of the body and how it works is concerned, breakfast is not a good idea for the following reasons: a) the body has been at rest all night, so why should we get up after the inactivity of sleep and put a big breakfast into the stomach? b) Big breakfasts drain and exhaust us of the energy that has been gathered in the night's sleep. c) Morning energy is the highest and represents the best potential for creative and physical work, for studying, writing, figuring, organizing. d) A meal requires most of the total nerve energy of the body to handle the digestion, and thus the mind becomes enervated, making us sluggish. e) It takes hours for the food eaten in breakfast to be processed before we gain any energy or vitality from it. Thus the idea that breakfast is the most important meal of the day, because it gives us the strength to do a hard morning's work, is false. Breakfast decreases the energy that we are able to bring to our morning's work because a lot of the fresh energy created by the night's sleep is requisitioned for the digestive process.

One of Bragg's rules of thumb is that we should earn the food we eat by physical activity. If we haven't done anything, we probably don't need another meal. It might be added that the hours of night represent a natural fasting time for the body, and going until noon before eating again extends the period of time in which our internal systems can accomplish their cleansing, restorative, and healing projects.

Arnold Ehret has a theory as to why, when we get up in the morning after having done no physical activity, we still want to eat. During the night, when our stomach has been free from food, the body starts the eliminating process as if it were on a mini-fast. When we wake up in the morning we feel miserable and have a coating on the tongue because the waste is already being released into the blood stream for elimination. Since it's the process of elimination that makes us feel sluggish, and since the only thing that stops this process is refilling the stomach with food, we have developed the habit of eating as a way of making ourselves feel better—even though our bodies don't need the food. He, by the way, doesn't eat breakfast, says he feels much better, works more efficiently, and enjoys his luncheon more than ever.

Dr. Stuart B. Hill, member of the Canada Health Science Council, has a different theory of why one wants to eat in the morning after having done no physical activity during the night. His theory, which focuses on allergies and their adaptive-addictive relationships, is based on more recent research and information. "People tend to like to eat the things that poison them," he said to me in a conversation. "We adjust our lives around our allergic foods so that we keep our corticoids (an adrenal mechanism that defends against specific poisons) high and in a stimulated state. Thus in the morning we are craving for stimulation from the foods to which we became sensitized in early childhood (wheat, milk, eggs, etc.)." This theory is more fully set forth in an unpublished report by Dr. Hill and Dr. Donald Mitchell, the latter a clinical ecologist who has been supervising fasts for people over twenty years.

Foods eaten daily are most commonly suspected of being the causes of health problems. These foods comprise such staples as eggs, wheat, potatoes, cow's milk, oranges, beef, peas, beans, sugar, tea and coffee. . . .

When the body is exposed repeatedly to a substance that it is sensitive to, the endocrine control system responds by increasing its capacity to produce the necessary stimulant hormones.... This prepares the body for a quick response to a further exposure to the particular substance or to others to which the body reacts in a similar way. Instead of discomfort, a sense of increased well-being now follows exposure. There is the tendency then to consider oneself to be no longer reactive rather than being more deeply involved, which is the true situation. . . .

Persons who have become aware of their particular "poisons" have found that they can enjoy nearly total health, so long as they vary their exposures and eliminate indicated substances....

A new way of living based on restriction must be learned for the enjoyment of total health.

Both doctors have become involved in fasting because one approach to testing for sensitivity has been to eliminate the suspected foods from the diet for a week or so and then to reintroduce them as single food meals, recording any symptoms and signs that arise, e.g., changes in pulse, temperature, blood pressure, respiration, flushing, sweating, fatigue, nasal discharge, sneezing, coughing, restlessness, etc. This procedure has been found to be more satisfactory after a fast of a few days.

Underweight. People are not nourished in proportion to the amount of food they eat, but in proportion to how much they digest and assimilate. Food and nutrition are not the same thing. The amount of food taken in is not the key to the state of nutrition; the key is how much food is digested and assimilated. When the organs of digestion and assimilation are in poor working condition, eating too many fatty foods to gain weight defeats its own purpose. The key to improving health through weight gain may lie in the direction of rendering the detoxifying system more effective through fasting. There's considerable evidence that fasting helps the chronically underweight person to repair his or her assimilation functions. This should be done under medical supervision, however. The point is that when underweight is due to impairment of the general health of the person, it is futile to stuff a lot of food into the body when assimilation and digestion are malfunctioning. It is precisely those systems that need to be rejuvenated. Ironically, abstaining from food for a period of time can actually help a person gain weight in the long run through providing a period of physiological rest. Since the bodily metabolism is improved by fasting, the fast assists the body to assimilate proteins, fats, carbohydrates, starches, sugars, minerals, vitamins and all essential nutrients necessary for the body to work efficiently.

Heart Problems. We hold the record. It's a dubious distinction but the people in our part of the world lead everyone else in heart and artery problems. Every second of the day someone is dying of a heart attack. Heart trouble is one of the scourges of Western civilization. Yet, diseases of the heart do not build up rapidly. It takes a long time to harden and block an artery. There are many contributing causes: cholesterol, fats, and fibrous tissues are responsible for the blocking and obstructing of the arteries; lack of exercise also contributes to arterial degeneration. As the inner passage of the arteries becomes so narrow that not enough blood can flow through to properly nourish the heart muscle, coronary occlusion occurs. One fine morning, someone you or I know who hs generally neglected to care for the gift of his or her health gets out of bed to start the day's activities and clutches at the heart. She or he either dies abruptly of a heart attack or has to live with a serious chronic condition the rest of his or her life. In the average person who eats the average diet of today, the blockage grows silently, and when the blood can no longer flow freely through the arteries, disaster strikes. "We are all as old as our arteries," Bragg says. Inasmuch as it is a cleanser of internal impurities, fasting represents preventive health care. The systematic practice of fasting can add years to our lives. Surely the Creator who has given us so precious a gift as life does not wish that we be reckless with it.

Stiff Joints. Where does the toxic residue go that is left in the body after years of over- or wrong-eating? Some of it is concentrated and crystalized and finds its way into the moveable joints in the body. If you roll your head around right now, you may hear a grating, grinding sound. What you hear is the grinding of the toxic acid crystals that have alkalified themselves on the first bone of the spine. The first place people are likely to notice them is in their feet because there are more moveable bones there (twenty-six) than any other part of the body, and the force of gravity helps them move in that direction. When these calcium-like spurs attach themselves on the joints, and calcified substances replace the synovial fluid, the aches and pains begin. When there are excess toxins in the body, it's open season on the joints: ankles, knees, hips, spine, shoulders, elbows, wrists, fingers. It takes time to break down the toxic crystals through fasting that we have accumulated over the years and to dispel much of them, but fasting supervisors claim it can be done. Our self-repairing, self-healing, and self-maintaining powers are amazing, and are part of the richness of the gift God has given us when he gave us ourselves. As we are shown in the parable of the talents, what is given is not meant to be buried in a field. It is meant to be used.

Premature Aging. It is widely claimed in the literature that the biological process of aging is slowed by systematic fasting. Herbert Shelton, a director of thousands of fasts, has reported on this phenomenon. It is the debris of the metabolic process (converting food into living matter, and the matter into energy) that brings on many of our physical miseries and causes premature aging. We need to eliminate that debris through the bowels, the kidneys, the lungs, and the skin. We need, in other words, to keep clean inside. This is the secret of health and long life. As we have seen, nature's method for purifying and rejuvenating our body-self is fasting.

Addictions. Once our bodies have become clean through fasting, our physiological systems will do their best to reject poisons. It sets up an active resistance to any new poisons that try to enter. People who have tried to break their addictions to coffee, alcohol, tobacco, or drugs have found fasting a great help in kicking the habit. If it doesn't taste or feel good, it's going to lose its attraction.

What Are They Saying About Fasting?

The literature turned out by the best-known clinicians of fasting (Cott, Bragg, Ehret, Buchinger) is replete with testimonial claims. The modern woman or man today, already disappointed too many times by formulas for health and happiness that never delivered, approaches such testimony with a healthy sense of skepticism. That is as it should be. What cannot be denied is that there is something to be dealt with here. And if it is to be affirmed or negated, there is no substitute for personal experience.

What are those who have tried it saying? Here's a summary:

You Feel Healthier. People have observed that after a few days of going without food they feel better physically, mentally, and spiritually. All this time the animals have been running around hoarding their little secret: fasting is therapeutic. When your dog or cat is sick, it stops eating. And all these years we've answered "I'm really not hungry" with "C'mon—you've got to eat something; it'll build up your resistance!" And then nausea and feelings of discomfort followed. *Because* we ate.

How can bears and woodchucks hibernate for months without a a morsel of food? How do birds and beasts of prey get along nicely without food for two weeks or longer? How can the energetic salmon journey upstream for thousands of miles to spawn without taking nourishment along the way? Because they have amazing resources of energy that they can draw upon during that fasting period. People who have habitually abused their bodies with too much food (and the wrong kinds) often testify after their first fast that they felt really well for the first time they could remember. "We are what we eat" doesn't refer just to our physical being—it refers to our mental health as well. The state of nutrition in our system affects our behavior and our mood (which means our sanity). Extrasensory instinct becomes very

142

keen through fasting. The fast sharpens the mind, attunes one more closely with the gentle voice of nature. The mind works more freshly and perceptively after each fast because fasting has the effect of making the inner mind more alert.

You Feel Tranquil. Fasting is simply restful. It's anxiety and tension relieving, sometimes downright exhilarating. We sometimes turn to eating because we're anxious. We don't really need the food, but having something to do and the taste of food provide us with grateful distraction for awhile. The aftermath of overeating, however, brings on fresh anxieties related to health. The last state of anxiety is worse than the first!

A mind-boggling 100 million (nearly half of the U.S. population) complain of difficulty in getting to and staying asleep. Fasting, nature's tranquilizer, relaxes the nervous system and eases the anxieties that account for much sleeplessness. It's what's going on in the internal organs that often keeps us awake; if they're at rest, sleep is going to flow much more naturally. Insomnia is directly related to overeating, heartburn, bloating, acid indigestion. A further bonus is that when the body is operating more efficiently (as is the case when one fasts regularly), many people find that they do not require as much sleep as they once did.

You Look and Feel Younger. Fasting is a detoxifying strategy that gives the system a "clean bill of health." We're absorbing poisons all the time from the food we eat and the air we breathe. Doctors who have supervised fasts say that with a fast of a week or so they can be flushed out. The internal disorders are frequently reflected externally. All kinds of skin disorders, for example, have been known to benefit from fasting. It isn't that the acne or exzema or psoriasis is cured by the fasting itself, but that abstention from food leads to a selective eating diet which discovers the foods or combinations of foods that are causing the trouble. Under the teenagers' myth that "I can't eat that chocolate or I'll get zits" lies the theory that skin irritations are often caused by habitual overeating, particularly of starches and sugars.

The health-improvement claims that one finds in the literature on fasting cover a wide range. Researchers have seen bald patients start to grow hair again after fasts of only ten days. Sufferers of such assorted ailments as constipation, hay fever, asthma, peptic ulcers, arthritis, and colitis witness that their symptoms were significantly alleviated or disappeared altogether after a fast. Yogis say fasting gives them increased agility and concentration (a full stomach doesn't want to think—or be twisted). Those who suffer from hay fever find the pollen seasons easier to take with regular fasting. Some people report that, after a fast, their skin takes on a better color and texture; eyes clear up and become brighter.

Dr. Cott presents an article in *Health* magazine which states unequivocally that if the average person were to fast one day out of every week for a whole year "he would be no older in body at the year's end than in the beginning." In India a seventy-six year-old political dissident, Tara Singh, undertook a highly publicized fast of forty-eight days. Examining physicians said afterward that in their opinion his abstention from food has increased his life span by ten years. And Mohandas K. Gandhi, at sixty-four, was told on the tenth day of a fast that he was physiologically as healthy as a man of forty.

Smoking and Drinking Is Worse, Sex Is Better. For the person who would like to drink and smoke less, fasting provides more supportive reasons to leave it right where it is: in the bottle and in the pack. Drinking alcoholic beverages on an empty stomach (especially when its going to stay empty for awhile) may make you very dizzy and nauseous. If fasting is approached from the point of body ecology, and nicotine and alcohol are seen as injecting more poisons into the system, the contradiction is obvious. One of the nice things about fasting is that as the body becomes purified there seems to be a built-in resistance toward polluting it all over again. The sense of well-being that accompanies fasting is a splendid opportunity to modify (dare it be said—give up) dependence on tobacco, alcohol, drugs, and pills. Regular fasting can clean out the taste buds and help one remember how bad that first cigarette or drink tasted.

Perhaps it is fasting's impact on weight loss that enhances sexual enjoyment in a couple of different ways. It's usually the case that when someone loses weight they feel better about themselves, they feel more attractive. They also have a lot more energy because the body isn't huffing and puffing under too much freight. Dr. Cott notes that many men and women attest that fasting made a qualitative difference in their sex life; for the first time there was a note of *vigor*. Some discovered that for the first time in their lives they felt sexually desirable.

You Save Time and Money. To look at the cost of groceries is bad enough, but to look at the cost of being sick is even worse (and, as has been demonstrated, the kind of groceries we buy and the way we consume them is frequently related to being sick). A lot of people are realizing that if they fast just one day a week, they will cut their food bill by 15 percent (to say nothing of the added benefits of keeping

144

their waste where they want it). Just skipping dinner one night a week cuts 5 percent off the food budget.

Certainly, eating is meant to be one of life's chief joys: A humane celebration of taste, color, smell and texture. When people sit down to table together, it should be an event that closes the door on routine and opens a new space and time in which the food that is passed from hand to hand becomes a symbol of deeper sharings among those around the table. It is meant to be a time when the art of conversation is learned, where laughter levels the anxieties of the day. The meal experience is meant to be more than just putting food into our bodies.

The sad truth for many moderns, however, is that it isn't. It's an on-the-run, catch-as-catch-can, put-some-fuel-in-the-tank-to-keep-yourself-going experience. It often becomes, unfortunately, sheer pragmatics, as is witnessed by the tremendous number of people sitting alone and staring out the window at passers-by from the stools and chairs of fast-food restaurants. Many are deciding that if that's all there is to lunch or supper—just food, minus any social sharing, they don't really need that hamburger. As a matter of fact, the time normally given to eating can be spent in other, more life-giving pursuits. "More life-giving," because three meals a day aren't necessarily what is healthiest. If we shifted from three meals a day to two, how many hours would that free up each week for something that may be more of a real need in our lives, like exercise or reading or prayer?

Real Virtue Is Attractive

The above are just some of the ways that fasting acts as a way of caring for, respecting, and loving ourselves. We begin life with such marvelous endowments that the Psalmist was moved to ask God, "What is man, that you have made him little less than the angels?" In our powers of intellect and will, God has given us what we need to comprehend our situation and to make choices that are life-supporting. He has given us built-in natural resources for health and healing. There are no short-cuts. Our internal systems are the original Big Brother (and Big Sister): every attempt to cheat is caught, and there's always a retribution.

Virtue is the power and readiness to do what is good, and that's what our situation calls for: The habit of doing what's good. Joyfully and perseveringly. Any way we cut it, that last characteristic is vital: perseverance, consistency.

A smile tugs at the corners of my mouth as I write these lines, because I can hear in my head some of my friends saying, "Yuuucch! How boring!" One of them used to tell me, "When I watch you going out to 'jock it up' every morning, the thought occasionally comes to me: 'Wouldn't you like to jog, or swim, or cross-country ski, too?' But then I recognize it as the temptation it is, and go into my room, pull the shades, get into bed, draw the covers over my head, and wait till it passes!"

I can hear that same voice bantering, "You go ahead and fight the good fight. Every army needs its standard bearers. As for me, I choose to *enjoy* my life. . . ."

That kind of teasing is like the song "Fie on Goodness!" from *Camelot*: on the one hand it makes us chuckle, and on the other, we identify with the yearning for comfort and indulgence, with the popular myth that wanton living is exciting and fulfilling, while virtuous living is dull and boring. Here are some of the lyrics:

> Fie on goodness! Fie!
> Eight years of kindness to your neighbor,
> making sure that the meek are treated well,
> Eight years of philanthropic labor,
> Darie down dell
> Gad, but it's hell! . . .
>
> It's been depressing all the way
> Darie down, darie down
> I'm getting glummer every day
> Darie down, darie down
> Anything to laugh again!
>
> When I think of the rollicking pleasures
> That earlier filled my life . . .
> Fie on goodness! Fie! . . .
>
> Lechery and vice have been arrested. . . .
> No one repents for any sin now,
> Every soul is immaculate and trim,
> No one is public with chagrin now. . . .
>
> There's not a folly to deplore
> Darie down, darie down

Confession Sunday is a bore,
Darie down, darie down,
Ah, but to spend a tortured evening
Staring at the floor,
Guilty and alive once more!

Fie on virtue, Fie!
Fie on goodness, Fie!

I'm sure one of the reasons I enjoy that song so much is that it touches something human in us and our experience: the attractiveness of "evil," the lure of the "forbidden." We're tempted to believe that virtue is for weaklings—not for the kind of people who smoke Marlboro and drink Canadian Club. Virtue's payoff oftentimes seems to be too far away to be worth the sacrifice. In an age of instant communication and fast-food restaurants, many have little patience for anything that does not show a profit immediately. The tendency today is to "hang loose" and not to tie ourselves to anything that may prove too costly, to "keep our options open."

But I don't think anyone who has ever given him or herself over to the unbridled pursuit of pleasure in an undisciplined life found that it delivered the kind of fulfillment promised or sought for. The truth is that a genuinely virtuous life is both immensely attractive and has a rich yield of what we all are looking for: inner peace and a deep, abiding joy. When we meet a truly virtuous person, we forget the insinuations and sentiments of the song from *Camelot*. When Pope John Paul II visited the United States in October of 1979, millions of people were drawn by his charisma. Said Rabbi Kelman, a Jewish leader in New York City: "All I know is that my son, Levi, a young rabbi who is going to Israel, attended the service in St. Patrick's Cathedral and said that he got tremendous spiritual vibrations from this man. I feel the same way. He has a tremendous love for people." The Rev. William Sloane Coffin, Presbyterian pastor of the Riverside Church in Manhattan, said he "felt a very deep humanity that speaks to our longing for genuine charity and wisdom." And Father Ellwood Kaiser, a Paulist priest from Los Angeles who has produced over 300 television dramas over the past twenty years, remarked, "He's a man's man, earthy . . . who symbolizes what a man can be when he surrenders his life to God."

There is a quality to the presence of a genuinely virtuous person that fascinates, invites, and challenges. When Vice President Mondale said good-bye to John Paul at the airport, he said: "You have unleashed the best and most generous sentiments within us, and given us courage to go forward." That's what virtue does.

Jesus was not a weak or unattractive human being for following the way of authentic virtue. He brought all his human powers and capacities to fulfillment as the Spirit prompted him. He was a fully alive and admiring human because he was loving, just, courageous, and humble.

The four basic virtues that Christian tradition gives us as the cornerstones for every other conceivable virtue are prudence, fortitude, temperance, and justice. They have been called "the cardinal virtues," from the Latin word, *cardo*, meaning "hinge." They are the four heavy-duty hinges from which all moral virtues hang.

I think the practice of fasting involves something from each of them. *Prudence* is the power of good judgment. As we've seen in this chapter, God has endowed us with a mind and will capable of comprehending and putting to use our natural and in-built resources for health and healing. But we're expected to do our part, to exercise good judgment.

Temperance means moderation. Perhaps two meals a day instead of three. A fast day each week. A proper, balanced diet. Eating just what we need and learning to leave the table before we're stuffed. All these represent temperance in action.

Justice is the virtue of rendering to everyone what is their due. In chapter 5 we discussed how fasting relates to social justice and the hungry of the world. Augustine's words: "Your privations will be fruitful if you provide for the needs of another. Certainly you have deprived your body, but to whom did you give that which you deprived yourself? Fast, then, in such a way that when another has eaten in your place you may rejoice in the meal you have taken. Then your offering will be received by God."

Fortitude is the capacity to act courageously, to endure difficulty. Just wait until someone comes along on your fast day with a box of French pastries from *La Patisserie Belge*. If you're possessed of the heroism to weather that, you'll do just fine! (My assistant has threatened to send the publisher a picture of me sitting on our patio talking about fasting to some friends while eating a French pastry! Unfortunately, the universal state of virtue described in *Camelot's* "Fie on Goodness!" is not an imminent threat.)

Before he received the stigmata, the marks of the passion of Jesus Christ, St. Francis of Assisi was very hard on his own body. He starved it and subjected it to severe penances. He drove himself to physical extremes of exhaustion. However, once he was touched by the Lord on Mt. La Verna and received the stigmata, he began to ask forgiveness of "Brother Ass" (as he had affectionately dubbed his bodily self) for punishing himself instead of embracing his being in its totality.

That is what spirituality today is asking us to do. To embrace God wherever he is, and God is "in," not simply "out there." He is in me, my body-spirit, in my neighbor, in my efforts to work for a just society, in my emotions and longings, in my struggle and joy, in my maleness or femaleness, in my fasting and my eating. This "way" of spiritual growth challenges us to find God where he is. When we find the Lord, and let him touch us, we are made whole. Holy.

Then, as St. Francis writes in his last testament, "what before seemed repulsive is turned into sweetness of soul" for us because of that loving, holy touch of the Lord. We move from an "I'm-a-mess" theology to an "I-love-what-I-see" theology. Because of that new attitude of self-love and self-acceptance, "instead of getting to heaven at last, we're going there all along!"

7 Appendix: Prayers for a Fast Day

Psalm 4:
Joyful Confidence in God

(I) When I call, answer me, O my just God,
    you who relieve me when I am in distress;
Have pity on me, and hear my prayer!

(II) Men of rank, how long will you be dull of heart?
    Why do you love what is vain and
      seek after falsehood?
Know that the Lord does wonders for
    his faithful one;
      the Lord will hear me when I call
upon him.
Tremble, and sin not;
    reflect, upon your beds, in silence.
Offer just sacrifices,
    and trust in the Lord.

(III) Many say, "Oh, that we might see better
    times!"
O Lord, let the light of your countenance
    shine upon us!
You put gladness into my heart,
    more than when grain and wine abound.
As soon as I lie down, I fall peacefully
    asleep,
      for you alone, O Lord,
bring security to my dwelling.

Psalm 16:
God the Supreme Good

(I) Keep me, O God, for in you I take
    refuge;
    I say to the Lord, "My Lord are you.

Apart from you I have no good."
How wonderfully has he made me
    cherish
    the holy ones who are in his land!
They multiply their sorrows
    who court other gods.
Blood libations to them I will not pour
    out,
        nor will I take their names upon
    my lips.
O Lord, my allotted portion and my
    cup,
    you it is who hold fast my lot.
For me the measuring lines have fallen
    on pleasant sites;
    fair to me indeed is my inheritance.

(II) I bless the Lord who counsels me;
        even in the night my heart exhorts
    me.
    I set the Lord ever before me;
        with him at my right hand I shall
    not be disturbed.
Therefore my heart is glad and my
    soul rejoices,
    my body, too, abides in confidence;
Because you will not abandon my soul
    to the nether world,
        nor will your suffer your faithful one
    to undergo corruption.
You will show me the path to life,
    fullness of joys in your presence,
    the delights at your right hand
    forever.

Psalm 63:
Ardent Longing for God

(I) O God, you are my God whom I seek;
    for you my flesh pines and my soul thirsts
    like the earth, parched, lifeless and
        without water.

Thus have I gazed toward you in the
    sanctuary
to see your power and your glory,
For your kindness is a greater good
    than life;
    my lips shall glorify you.

(II) Thus will I bless you while I live;
    lifting up my hands, I will call upon
    your name.
As with the riches of a banquet shall
    my soul be satisfied,
    and with exultant lips my mouth
    shall praise you.
I will remember you upon my couch,
    and through the night-watches I will
    meditate on you:
That you are my help,
    and in the shadow of your wings I
    shout for joy.

My soul clings fast to you;
    your right hand upholds me.

Psalm 71:
Humble Prayer

(I) In you, O Lord, I take refuge;
    let me never be put to shame.
In your justice rescue me, and deliver me;
    incline your ear to me, and save me.
Be my rock of refuge,
    a stronghold to give me safety,
    for you are my rock and my fortress.
O my God, rescue me from the hand
    of the wicked,
    from the grasp of the criminal and
    the violent.
For you are my hope, O Lord;
    my trust, O God, from my youth.
On you I depend from birth;

from my mother's womb you are my
    strength;
    constant has been my hope in you.
A sign of contradiction am I to many,
    but you are my strong refuge!
My mouth shall be filled with your praise,
    with your glory day by day.

Psalm 91:
Security under God's Protection

You who dwell in the shelter of the
        Most High,
    who abide in the shadow of the
        Almighty,
Say to the Lord, "My refuge and my
        fortress,
    my God, in whom I trust."
For he will rescue you from the snare
        of the fowler,
    from the destroying pestilence,
With his pinions he will cover you,
    and under his wings you shall take
        refuge;
    his faithfulness is a buckler and a
        shield.
You shall not fear the terror of the
        night
    nor the arrow that flies by day:
Not the pestilence that roams in darkness
    nor the devastating plague at noon.
Though a thousand fall at your side,
    ten thousand at your right side,
    near you it shall not come.
Rather with your eyes shall you behold
    and see the requital of the wicked,
Because you have the Lord for your
        refuge;
    you have made the Most HIgh your
        stronghold.

Psalm 102:
Prayer in Time of Distress

(I) O Lord, hear my prayer,
    and let my cry come to you.
Hide not your face from me
    in the day of my distress.
Incline your ear to me;
    in the day when I call, answer
    me speedily.
For my days vanish like smoke,
    and my bones burn like fire.
Withered and dried up like grass is
    my heart;
    I forget to eat my bread.
Because of my insistent sighing
    I am reduced to skin and bone.
I am like a desert owl;
    I have become like an owl among
    the ruins.
I am sleepless, and I moan;
    I am like a sparrow alone on the
    the housetop.
All the day my enemies revile me;
    in their rage against me they make
    a curse of me.
For I eat ashes like bread
    and mingle my drink with tears,
Because of your fury and your wrath;
    for you lifted me up only to cast me
    down.
My days are like a lengthening
    shadow,
    and I wither like grass.

(II) But you, O Lord, abide forever,
    and your name through all generations.
You will arise and have mercy on Zion,
    for it is time to pity her,
    for the appointed time has come.

Psalm 103:
Praise of Divine Goodness

(I) Bless the Lord, O my soul;
　　and all my being, bless his holy name.
　Bless the Lord, O my soul,
　　and forget not all his benefits;
　He pardons all your iniquities,
　　he heals all your ills.
　He redeems your life from destruction,
　　he crowns you with kindness and compassion,
　He fills your lifetime with good;
　　your youth is renewed like the eagle's.

(II) The Lord secures justice
　　and the rights of all the oppressed.
　He has made known his ways to Moses,
　　and his deeds to the children of Israel.
　Merciful and gracious is the Lord,
　　slow to anger and abounding in kindness.
　He will not always chide,
　　nor does he keep his wrath forever.
　Not according to our sins does he deal with us,
　　Nor does he requite us according to our crimes.

(III) For as the heavens are high above the earth,
　　so surpassing is his kindness toward those who fear him.
　As far as the east is from the west,
　　so far has he put our transgressions from us.
　As a father has compassion on his children,
　　so the Lord has compassion on those who fear him,
　For he knows how we are formed;
　　he remembers that we are dust.
　Man's days are like those of grass;
　　like a flower of the field he blooms;
　The wind sweeps over him and he is gone,
　　and his place knows him no more.
　But the kindness of the Lord is from eternity
　　to eternity toward those who fear him,
　And his justice toward children's children
　　among those who keep his covenant
　　and remember to fulfill his precepts.

155

(IV) The Lord has established his throne in heaven,
and his kingdom rules over all.
Bless the Lord, all you his angels,
you mighty in strength, who do his bidding,
obeying his spoken word.
Bless the Lord, all you his hosts,
his ministers, who do his will.
Bless the Lord, all his works,
everywhere in his domain.
Bless the Lord, O my soul!

Psalm 111:
Praise of God for His Goodness

I will give thanks to the Lord with all my heart
in the company and assembly of the just.
Great are the works of the Lord,
exquisite in all their delights.
Majesty and glory are his work,
and his justice endures forever.
He has won renown for his wondrous deeds;
gracious and merciful is the Lord.
He has given food to those who fear him;
he will forever be mindful of his covenant.
He has made known to his people the power of his works,
giving them the inheritance of the nations.
The works of his hands are faithful and just;
sure are all his precepts,
Reliable forever and ever,
wrought in truth and equity.
He has sent deliverance to his people;
he has ratified his covenant forever;
holy and awesome is his name.
The fear of the Lord is the beginning of wisdom;
prudent are all who live by it.
His praise endures forever.

Psalm 138:
Hymn of a Grateful Heart

(I) I will give thanks to you, O Lord, with all my heart,
(for you have heard the words of my mouth);

FOR FURTHER READING

Books

Buchinger, Otto. *Everything You Want to Know about Fasting.* New York: Pyramid Books, 1972.

Cott, Allan. *Fasting as a Way of Life.* New York: Bantam Books, 1977.

Cott, Allan. *Fasting: The Ultimate Diet.* New York: Bantam Books, 1975.

Farrell, Walter. *A Companion to the Summa.* Vol. III: *The Fullness of Life.* New York: Sheed and Ward, 1940.

Knowles, David and Dimitry Obolensky. *The Middle Ages.* New York: McGraw-Hill, 1968.

Simon, Arthur. *Bread for the World.* New York: Paulist Press, 1975.

Smuts, J. C. *Holism and Evolution.* London: Macmillan, 1926.

Van Kaam, Adrian and Susan Muto. *Am I Living a Spiritual Life?* Denville, N.J.: Dimension Books, 1978.

Weil, Andrew. *The Natural Mind.* Boston, Houghton Mifflin, 1972.

Periodicals

"For God's Sake, Fast for Your Own Sake," *Christian Century* (February 28, 1968).

Jones, Susan Smith. "The Valuable Art of Fasting," *Runner's World* (June, 1978).

Maloney, George A. "Following Jesus in the Real World," *Asceticism Today*, 1979.

Marin, Peter. "The New Narcissism," *Harper's Magazine* (October, 1975).

Wolf, Linda and Dr. Otto Kernberg. "Why Some People Can't Love," *Psychology Today* (June, 1978).